A Handbook of Health

by Woods Hutchinson

PREFACE

Looking upon the human body from the physical point of view as the most perfect, most ingeniously economical, and most beautiful of living machines, the author has attempted to write a little handbook of practical instruction for the running of it.

And seeing that, like other machines, it derives the whole of its energy from its fuel, the subject of foods--their properties, uses, and methods of preparation--has been gone into with unusual care. An adequate supply of clean-burning food-fuel for the human engine is so absolutely fundamental both for health and for efficiency--we are so literally what we have eaten-- that to be well fed is in very fact two-thirds of the battle of life from a physiological point of view. The whole discussion is in accord with the aim, kept in view throughout the book, of making its suggestion and advice positive instead of negative, pointing out that, in the language of the old swordsman, "attack is the best defense." If we actively do those things that make for health and efficiency, and which, for the most part, are attractive and agreeable to our natural instincts and unspoiled tastes,--such as exercising in the open air, eating three square meals a day of real food, getting nine or ten hours of undisturbed sleep, taking plenty of fresh air and cold water both inside and out,--this will of itself carry us safely past all the forbidden side paths without the need of so much as a glance at the "Don't" and "Must not" with which it has been the custom to border and fence in the path of right living.

On the other hand, while fully alive to the undesirability, and indeed wickedness, of putting ideas of dread and suffering into children's minds unnecessarily, yet so much of the misery in the world is due to ignorance, and could have been avoided if knowledge of the simplest character had been given at the proper time, that it has been thought best to set forth the facts as to the causation and nature of the commonest diseases, and the methods by which they may be avoided. This is peculiarly necessary from the fact that most of the gravest enemies of mankind have come into existence within a comparatively recent period of the history of life,--only since the beginning of civilization, in fact,--so that we have as yet developed no natural instincts for their avoidance.

Nor do we admit that we are adding anything to the stock of fears in the minds of children--the nurse-maid and the bad boys in the next alley have been ahead of us in this respect. The child-mind is too often already filled with fears and superstitions of every sort, passed down from antiquity. Modern sanitarians have been accused of merely substituting one fear for another in the mind of the child--bacilli instead of bogies. But, even if this be true, there are profound and practical differences between the two terrors. One is real, and the other imaginary. A child cannot avoid meeting a bacillus; he will never actually make the acquaintance of a bogie. Children, like savages and ignorant adults, believe and invent and retail among themselves the most extraordinary and grotesque theories about the structure and functions of their bodies, the nature and causation of their illnesses and aches and pains. A plain and straightforward statement of the actual facts about these things not only will not shock or repel them, or make them old before their time, but, on the contrary, will interest them greatly, relieve their minds of many unfounded dreads, and save them from the commonest and most hurtful mistakes of humanity--those that are committed through ignorance.

THE AUTHOR.

CONTENTS

A HANDBOOK OF HEALTH

CHAPTER I

RUNNING THE HUMAN AUTOMOBILE

The Body-Automobile. If you were to start to-morrow morning on a long-distance ride in an automobile, the first thing that you would do would be to find out just how that automobile was built; how often it must have fresh gasoline; how its different speed gears were worked; what its tires were made of; how to mend them; and how to cure engine troubles. To attempt to run an automobile, for even a ten-mile ride, with less information than this, would be regarded as foolhardy.

Yet most of us are willing to set out upon the journey of life in the most complicated, most ingenious, and most delicate machine ever made--our body--with no more knowledge of its structure than can be gained from gazing in the looking-glass; or of its needs, than a preference for filling up its fuel tank three times a day. More knowledge than this is often regarded as both unnecessary and unpleasant. Yet there are few things more important, more vital to our health, our happiness, and our success in life, than to know how to steer and how to road-repair our body-automobile. This we can learn only from physiology and hygiene.

The General Plan of the Human Automobile is Simple. Complicated as our body-automobile looks to be, there are certain things about the plan and general build of it which are plain enough. It has a head end, where fuel supplies are taken in and where its lamps and other look-out apparatus are carried; a body in which the fuel is stored and turned into work or speed, and into which air is drawn to help combustion and to cool the engine pipes. It has a pair of fore-wheels (the arms) and a pair of hind-wheels (the legs), though these have been reduced to only one spoke each, and swing only about a quarter of the way around and back again when running, instead of round and round. It has a steering gear (the brain), just back of the headlights, and a system of nerve electric wires connecting all parts of it. It gets warm when it runs, and stops if it is not fed.

There is not an unnecessary part, or unreasonable "cog," anywhere in the whole of our bodies. It is true that there are a few little remnants which are not quite so useful as they once were, and which sometimes cause trouble. But for the most part, all we have to do is to look long and carefully enough at any organ or part of our bodies, to be able to puzzle out just what it is or was intended to do, and why it has the shape and size it has.

Why the Study of Physiology is Easy. There is one thing that helps to make the study of physiology quite easy. It is that you already know a good deal about your body, because you have had to live with it for a number of years past, and you can hardly have helped becoming somewhat acquainted with it during this time.

You have, also, another advantage, which will help you in this study. While your ideas of how to take care of your body are rather vague, and some of them wrong, most of them are in the main right, or at least lead you in the right direction. You all know enough to eat when you are hungry and to drink when you are thirsty, even though you don't always know when to stop, or just what to eat. You like sunny days better than cloudy ones, and would much rather breathe fresh air than foul. You like to go wading and swimming when you are hot and dusty, and you don't need to be told to go to sleep when you are tired. You would much rather have sugar than vinegar, sweet milk than sour milk; and you dislike to eat or drink anything that looks dirty or foul, or smells bad.

These inborn likes and dislikes--which we call instincts--are the forces which have built up this wonderful body-machine of ours in the past and, if properly understood and trained, can be largely trusted to run it in the future. How to follow these instincts intelligently, where to check them, where to encourage them, how to keep the proper balance between them, how to live long and be useful and happy--this is what the interesting study of physiology and hygiene will teach you.

CHAPTER II

WHY WE HAVE A STOMACH

WHAT KEEPS US ALIVE

The Energy in Food and Fuel. The first question that arises in our mind on looking at an engine or machine of any sort is, What makes it go? If we can succeed in getting an answer to the question, What makes the human automobile go? we shall have the key to half its secrets at once. It is fuel, of course; but what kind of fuel? How does the body take it in, how does it burn it, and how does it use the energy or power stored up in it to run the body-engine?

Man is a bread-and-butter-motor. The fuel of the automobile is gasoline, and the fuel of the man-motor we call food. The two kinds of fuel do not taste or smell much alike; but they are alike in that they both have what we call energy, or power, stored up in them, and will, when set fire to, burn, or explode, and give off this power in the shape of heat, or explosions, which will do work.

Food and Fuel are the Result of Life. Fuels and foods are also alike in another respect; and that is, that, no matter how much they may differ in appearance and form, they are practically all the result of life. This is clear enough as regards our foods, which are usually the seeds, fruits, and leaves of plants, and the flesh of animals. It is also true of the cord-wood and logs that we burn in our stoves and fireplaces. But what of coal and gasoline? They are minerals, and they come, as we know, out of the depths of the earth. Yet they too are the product of life; for the layers of coal, which lie sixty, eighty, one hundred and fifty feet below the surface of the earth, are the fossilized remains of great forests and jungles, which were buried millions of years ago, and whose leaves and branches and trunks have been pressed and baked into coal. Gasoline comes from coal oil, or petroleum, and is simply the "juice" which was squeezed out of these layers of trees and ferns while they were being crushed and pressed into coal.

How the Sun is Turned into Energy by Plants and Animals. Where did the flowers and fruits and leaves that we now see, and the trees and ferns that grew millions of years ago, get this power, part of which made them grow and part of which was stored away in their leaves and branches and seeds? From the one place that is the source of all the force and energy and power in this world, the sun.

That is why plants will, as you know, flourish and grow strong and green only in the sunlight, and why they wilt and turn pale in the dark. When the plant grows, it is simply sucking up through the green stuff (chlorophyll) in its leaves the heat and light of the sun and turning it to its own uses. Then this sunlight, which has been absorbed by plants and built up into their leaves, branches, and fruits, and stored away in them as energy or power, is eaten by animals; and they in turn use it to grow and move about with.

Plants can use this sun-power only to grow with and to carry out a few very limited movements, such as turning to face the sun, reaching over toward the light, and so on. But animals, taking this power at second-hand from plants by eating their leaves or fruits, can use it not merely to grow with, but also to run, to fight, to climb, to cry out, and to carry out all those movements and processes which we call life.

Plants, on the other hand, are quite independent of animals; for they can take up, or drink, this sun-power directly, with the addition of water from the soil sucked up through their roots, and certain salts[1] melted in it. Plants can live, as we say, upon non-living foods. But animals must take their supply of sun-power at second-hand by eating the leaves and the fruits and the seeds of plants; or at third-hand by eating other animals.

All living things, including ourselves, are simply bundles of sunlight, done up in the form of cabbages, cows, and kings; and so it is quite right to say that a healthy, happy child has a "sunny" disposition.

Plants and Animals Differ in their Way of Taking Food. As plants take in their sun-food and their air directly through their leaves, and their drink of salty water through their roots, they need no special opening for the purpose of eating and drinking, like a mouth; or place for storing food, like a stomach. They have mouths and stomachs all over them, in the form of tiny pores on their leaves, and hair-like tubes sticking out from their roots. They can eat with every inch of their growing surface.

But animals, that have to take their sun-food or nourishment at second-hand, in the form of solid pieces of seeds, fruits, or leaves of plants, and must take their drink in gulps, instead of soaking it up all over their surface, must have some sort of intake opening, or mouth, somewhere on the surface; and some sort of pouch, or stomach, inside the body, in which their food can be stored and digested, or melted down. By this means they also get rid of the necessity of staying rooted in one place, to suck up moisture and food from the soil. One of the chief and most striking differences between plants and animals is that animals have mouths and stomachs, while plants have not.

THE DIGESTIVE SYSTEM

How the Food Reaches the Stomach. Our body, then, has an opening, which we call the mouth, through which our food-fuel can be taken in. A straight delivery tube, called the gullet, or esophagus, runs down from the mouth to a bag, or pouch, called the stomach, in which the food is stored until it can be used to give energy to the body, just as the gasoline is stored in the automobile tank until it can be burned.

The mouth opening is furnished with lips to open and close it and assist in picking up our food and in sucking up our drink; and, as much of our food is in solid form, and as the stomach can take care only of fluid and pulpy materials, nature has provided a mill in the mouth in the form of two arches, of semicircles, of teeth, which grind against each other and crush the food into a pulp.

In the bottom or floor of the mouth, there has grown up a movable bundle of muscles, called the tongue, which acts as a sort of waiter, handing the food about the mouth, pushing it between the teeth, licking it out of the pouches of the cheeks to bring it back into the teeth-mill again, and finally, after it has been reduced to a pulp, gathering it up into a little ball, or bolus, and shooting it back down the throat, through the gullet, into the stomach.

The Intestines. When the food has been sufficiently melted and partially digested in the stomach, it is pushed on into a long tube called the intestine, or bowel. During its passage through this part of the food tube, it is taken up into the veins, and carried to the heart. From here it is pumped all over the body to feed and nourish the millions of little cells of which the body is built. This bowel tube, or intestine, which, on account of its length, is arranged in coils, finally delivers the undigested remains of the food into a somewhat larger tube called the large intestine, in the lower and back part of the body, where its remaining moisture is sucked out of it, and its solid waste material passed out of the body through the rectum in the form of the feces.

THE JOURNEY DOWN THE FOOD TUBE

The Flow of Saliva and "Appetite Juice." We are now ready to start some food-fuel, say a piece of bread, on its journey down our food tube, or alimentary canal. One would naturally suppose that the process of digestion would not begin until the food got well between our teeth; but, as a matter of fact, it begins before it enters our lips, or even before it leaves the table. If bread be toasted or freshly baked, the mere smell of it will start our mouths to watering; nay, even the mere sight of food, as in a pastry cook's window, with the glass between us and it, will start up this preparation for the feast.

This flow of saliva in the mouth is of great assistance in moistening the bread while we are chewing it; but it goes farther than this. Some of the saliva is swallowed before we begin to eat; and this goes down into the stomach and brings word to the juices there to be ready, for something is coming. As the food approaches the mouth, a message also is telegraphed down the nerves to the stomach, which at once actively sets to work pouring out a digestive juice in readiness, called the "appetite juice." This shows how important are, not merely a good appetite, but also attractive appearance and flavor in our food; for if this appetite juice is not secreted, the food may lie in the stomach for hours before the proper process of digestion, or melting, begins.

The Salivary Glands. Now, where does this saliva in the mouth come from? It is poured out from the pouches of the cheeks, and from under the tongue, by some little living sponges, or juice factories, known as salivary glands.[2]

All the juices poured out by these glands, indeed nearly all the fluids or juices in our bodies, are either acid or alkaline. By acid we mean sour, or sharp, like vinegar, lemon juice, vitriol (sulphuric acid), and carbonic acid (which forms the bubbles in and gives the sharp taste to plain soda-water). By alkaline we mean "soap-like" or flat, like soda, lye, lime, and soaps of all sorts. If you pour an acid and an alkali together--like vinegar and soda--they will "fizz" or effervesce, and at the same time neutralize or "kill" each other.

The Use of the Saliva. As the chief purpose of digestion is to prepare the food so that it will dissolve in water, and then be taken up by the cells lining the food-tube, the saliva, like the rest of the body juices, consists chiefly of water. Nothing is more disagreeable than to try to chew some dry food--like a large, crisp soda cracker, for instance--which takes more moisture than the salivary glands are able to pour out on such short notice. You soon begin to feel as if you would choke unless you could get a drink of water. But it is not altogether advisable to take this short cut to relief, because the salivary juice contains what the drink of water does not--a ferment, or digestive substance (ptyalin), which possesses the power of turning the starch in our food into sugar. As starch is only very slowly soluble, or "meltable," in water, while sugar is very readily so, the saliva is of great assistance in the process of melting, known as digestion. The changing of the starch to sugar is the reason why bread or cracker, after it has been well chewed, begins to taste sweetish.

This change in the mouth, however, is not of such great importance as we at one time thought, because even with careful mastication, a certain amount of starch will be swallowed unchanged. Nature has provided for this by causing another gland farther down the canal, just beyond the stomach, called the pancreas, to pour into the food tube a juice which is far stronger in sugar-making power than the saliva, and this will readily deal with any starch which may have escaped this change in the mouth. Moreover, this "sugaring" of starch goes on in the stomach for twenty to forty minutes after the food has been swallowed.

Starchy foods, like bread, biscuit, crackers, cake, and pastry, are really the only ones which require such thorough and elaborate chewing as we sometimes hear urged. Other kinds of food, like meat and eggs--which contain no starch and consequently are not acted upon by the saliva--need be chewed only sufficiently long and thoroughly to break them up and reduce them to a coarse pulp, so that they can be readily acted upon by the acid juice of the stomach.

Down the Gullet. When the food has been thoroughly moistened and crushed in the mouth and rolled into a lump, or bolus, at the back of the tongue, it is started down the elevator shaft which we call the gullet, or esophagus. It does not fall of its own weight, like coal down a chute, but each separate swallow is carried down the whole nine inches of the gullet by a wave of muscular action. So powerful and closely applied is this muscular pressure that jugglers can train themselves, with practice, to swallow standing on their heads and even to drink a glass of water in that position; while a horse or a cow always drinks "up-hill." This driving power of the food tube extends throughout its entire length; it is carried out by a series of circular rings of muscles, which are bound together by other threads of muscle running lengthwise, together forming the so-called muscular coat of the tube. By contracting, or squeezing down in rapid succession, one after another, they move the food along through the tube. The failure of these little muscles to act properly is one of the causes of constipation and biliousness. Sometimes the action of the muscles is reversed, and then we get a gush of acid, or bitter, half-digested food up into the mouth, which we call "heart-burn" or "water-brash."

The Stomach--its Shape, Position, and Size. By means of muscular contraction, then, the gullet-elevator carries the food into the stomach. This is a comparatively simple affair, merely a ballooning out, or swelling, of the food tube, like the bulb of a syringe, making a pouch, where the food can be stored between meals, and where it can undergo a certain kind of melting or dissolving. This pouch is about the shape of a pear, with its larger end upward and pointing to the left, and its smaller end tapering down into the intestine, or bowel, on the right, just under the liver. The middle part of the stomach lies almost directly under what we call the "pit of the stomach," though far the larger part of it lies above and to the left of this point, going right up under the ribs until it almost touches the heart, the diaphragm only coming between.[3] This is one of the reasons why, when we have an attack of indigestion, and the stomach is distended with gas, we are quite likely to have palpitation and shortness of breath as well, because the gas-swollen left end of the stomach is pressing upward against the diaphragm and thus upon the heart and the lungs. Most cases of imagined heart trouble are really due to indigestion.

The Lining Surface of the Stomach. Now let us look more carefully at the lining surface of the stomach, for it is very wonderful. Like all other living surfaces, it consists of tiny, living units, or "body bricks" called cells, packed closely side by side like bricks in a pavement. We speak of the mucous membrane, or lining, of our food tube, as if it were one continuous sheet, like a piece of calico or silk; but we must never forget that it is made up of living ranks of millions of tiny cells standing shoulder to shoulder.

These cells are always actively at work picking out the substances they need, and manufacturing out of them the ferments and acids, or alkalies, needed for acting upon the food in their particular part of the tube, whether it be the mouth, the stomach, or the small intestine.

The Peptic Juice. The cells of the stomach glands manufacture and pour out a slightly sour, or acid, juice containing a ferment called pepsin. The acid, which is known as hydrochloric acid, and the pepsin together are able to melt down pieces of meat, egg, or curds of milk, and dissolve them into a clear, jelly-like fluid, or thin soup, which can readily be absorbed by the cells lining the intestine.[4]

You can see now why you shouldn't take large doses of soda or other alkalies, just because you feel a little uncomfortable after eating. They will make your stomach less acid and perhaps relieve the discomfort, but they stop or slow down digestion. Neither is it well to swallow large quantities of ice-water, or other very cold drinks, at meal times, or during the process of digestion. As digestion is largely getting the food dissolved in water, the drinking of moderate quantities of water, or other fluids, at meals is not only no hindrance, but rather a help in the process. The danger comes only when the drink is taken so cold as to check digestion, or when it is used to wash down the food in chunks, before it has been properly ground by the teeth.

The long duct of each gland is but a deep fold of the stomach lining (see note, p. 11). Into this duct the ranks of cells around it pour out the peptic juice.]

Digestion in the Stomach. Although usually a single, pear-shaped pouch, the stomach, during digestion, is practically divided into two parts by the shortening, or closing down, of a ring of circular muscle fibres about four inches from the lower end, throwing it into a large, rounded pouch on the left, and a small, cone-shaped one on the right. The gullet, of course, opens into the large left-hand pouch; and here the food is stored as it is swallowed until it has become sufficiently melted and acidified (mixed with acid juice) to be ready to pass on into the smaller pouch. Here more acid juice is poured out into it, and it is churned by the muscles in the walls of the stomach until it is changed to a jelly-like substance.

Digestion in the Small Intestine. The food-pulp now passes on into the small intestine, where it is acted upon by two other digestive juices--the bile, which comes from the liver, and the pancreatic juice, which is secreted by the pancreas.

The liver and the pancreas are a pair of large glands which have budded out, one on each side of the food tube, about six inches below where the food enters the small intestine from the stomach. The liver[5] weighs nearly three pounds, and the pancreas about a quarter of a pound.

Of these two glands, the pancreas, though the smaller, is far more important in digestion. In fact, it is the most powerful digestive gland in the body. Its juice, the pancreatic juice, can do everything that any other digestive juice can, and do it better. It contains a ferment for turning starch into sugar, which is far more powerful than that of the saliva; also another (trypsin), which will dissolve meat-stuffs nearly twice as fast as the pepsin of the stomach can; and still another, not possessed by either mouth or stomach glands, which will melt fat, so that it can be sucked up by the lining cells of the intestine.

What does this great combination of powers in the pancreas mean? It means that we have now reached the real centre and chief seat of digestion, namely, the small intestine, or upper bowel. This is where the food is really absorbed, taken up into the blood, and distributed to the body. All changes before this have been merely preparatory; all after it are simply a picking up of the pieces that remain.

In general appearance, this division of the food tube is very simple--merely a tube about twenty feet long and an inch in diameter, thrown into coils, so as to pack into small space, and slung up to the backbone by broad loops of a delicate tissue (mesentery). It looks not unlike twenty feet of pink garden hose.

The intestine also is provided with glands that pour out a juice known as the intestinal juice, which, although not very active in digestion, helps to melt down still further some of the sugars, and helps to prevent putrefaction, or decay, of the food from the bacteria[6] which swarm in this part of the tube.

By the time the food has gone a third of the way down the small intestine, a good share of the starches in it have been turned into sugar and absorbed by the blood vessels in its wall; and the meats, milk, eggs, and similar foods have been digested in the same way.

There still remains the bulk of the fats to be disposed of. These fats are attacked by the pancreatic juice and the bile, and made ready for digestion. Like other foods, they are then eaten by the cells of the intestinal wall; but instead of going directly into the blood vessels, as the sugars and other food substances do, they are passed on into another set of little tubes or vessels, called the lymphatics. In these they are carried through the lymph glands of the abdomen into the great lymph duct, which finally pours them into one of the great veins not far from the heart. Tiny, branching lymphatic tubes are found all over the body, picking up what the cells leave of the fluid which has seeped out of the arteries for their use and returning it to the veins through the great lymph duct.

All these different food substances, in the process of digestion, do not simply soak through the lining cells of the food tube, as through a blotting paper or straining cloth, but are actually eaten by the cells and very much changed in the process, and are then passed through the other side of the cells, either into the blood vessels of the wall of the intestine or into the lymph vessels, practically ready for use by the living tissues of the body. It is in the cells then that our food is turned into blood, and it is there that what we have eaten becomes really a part of us. It may even be said that we are living upon the leavings of the little cell citizens that line our food tube; but they are wonderfully decent, devoted little comrades of the rest of our body cells, and generous in the amount of food they pass on to the blood vessels.

As the food-pulp is squeezed on from one coil to another through the intestine, it naturally has more and more of its nourishing matter sucked out of it; until, by the time it reaches the last loop of the twenty feet of the small intestine, it has lost over two-thirds of its food value.

The Final Stage--the Journey through the Large Intestine. From the small intestine what remains of the food-pulp is poured into the last section of the food tube, which enlarges to from two to three inches in diameter. It is known as the large intestine, or large bowel. This section is only about five feet long. The first three-fourths of it is called the colon; the last or lowest quarter, the rectum, the discharge-pipe of the food tube. The principal use of the colon is to suck out the remaining traces of nourishing matter from the food and the water in which it is dissolved, thus gradually drying the food-pulp down to a solid or pasty form, in which condition it collects in a large "S" shaped loop of the bowel just above the rectum, until discharged.

The Waste Materials. By the time that the remains of the food-pulp have reached the middle of the large intestine, they have lost all their nutritive value and most of their water. All the way down from the upper part of the small intestine they have been receiving solid waste substances poured out by the glands of the intestines; indeed, the bulk of the feces is made up of these intestinal secretions, not, as is generally supposed, of the undigested remains of the food. Ninety-five per cent of our food is absorbed; the body-engine burns up its fuel very clean. The next largest part of the feces is bacteria, or germs; and the third and smallest, the indigestible fragments and remainders of food, such as vegetable fibres, bran, fruit skins, pits, seeds, etc. Hence the feces are not only worthless from a food point of view, but full of all sorts of possibilities for harm; and the principal interest of the body lies in getting rid of them as promptly and regularly as possible.

It can easily be seen how important it is that a habit should be formed, which nothing should be allowed to break, of promptly and regularly getting rid of these waste materials. For most persons, once in twenty-four hours is normal; for some, twice or even three times in the day. Whatever interval is natural, it should be attended to, beginning at a fixed hour every morning.

Constipation, and how to Prevent It. Constipation should not be treated by the all too common method of swallowing salts, which will cause a flood of watery matters to be poured through the food tube and sluice it clean of both poisons and melting food at the same time, leaving it in an exhausted and disturbed condition afterwards; nor by taking some irritating vegetable cathartic, generally in the form of pills, which sets up a violent action of the muscles of the food tube, driving its contents through at headlong speed; nor by washing out the lower two or three feet of the bowel with injections of water; although any or all of these may be resorted to occasionally for temporary relief. A very large portion of the food eaten is sucked out of the food tube into the blood vessels, passes through a large area of the body, and is poured out again as waste through the glands of the lining of the lower third of the bowel. Constipation, therefore, is caused by disturbances which interfere with these processes all over the body, not only in the stomach and bowels. Its only real and permanent cure is through exercise in the open air, sleep, and proper ventilation of bedrooms, with abundance of nourishing food, including plenty of green vegetables and fresh fruits.

The Appendix and Appendicitis. The beginning of the large bowel, where the small bowel empties into it, is the largest part of it, and forms a curious pouch called the cecum, or "blind" pouch. From one side of this projects a little wormlike tube, twisted and coiled upon itself, from three to six inches long and of about the size of a slate pencil. This is the famous appendix vermiformis (meaning, "wormlike tag"), which is such a frequent source of trouble. It is the shrunken and shriveled remains of a large pouch of the intestine which once opened into the cecum, and was used originally as a sort of second stomach for delaying and digesting the remains of the food. The reason why it gives rise to so much trouble is that it is so small--scarcely larger than will admit a knitting-needle--and so twisted upon itself that germs or other poisonous substances swallowed with the food may get into it, start a swelling or inflammation, get trapped in there by the closing of the narrow mouth of the tube, and form an abscess, which leaks through, or bursts into, the cavity of the body, called the peritoneum. This causes a very serious and often fatal blood poisoning.

Fortunately, appendicitis, or inflammation of the appendix, is not a very common disease, causing only one in one hundred of all deaths that occur; and these are mostly cases that were not treated promptly. Yet, if you have a severe, constant pain, rather low down in the right-hand corner of your abdomen, and if, when you press your hand firmly down in that corner, it hurts, or you feel a lump, it is decidedly safest to call a doctor and let him see what the condition really is, and advise you what to do.

FOOTNOTES:

[1] The term salts includes, as will be explained later, a large number of substances, like ordinary table salt, baking soda, and the laxative salts.

[2] There are three pairs of these: one just below the ears and behind the angles of the jaw, known as the parotid; one under the middle of the lower jaw known as the submaxillary; and a small pair just under the tip of the tongue, called the sublingual. These glands have grown up from the very simplest of beginnings. At first there was just a little pocketing or pouching down of the mucous lining, like the finger of a glove; then a couple of smaller hollow fingers budded off from the bottom of the first finger; then four smaller fingers from the bottom of these; and so on, until a regular little hollow tree or shrub of these tiny tubes was built up, all discharging through the original hollow stem, which has now become what we call the duct of the gland. Every secreting gland in the body--the stomach (or peptic) glands, the salivary glands, the liver, the pancreas--is built up upon this simple plan. The saliva and the juice of the pancreas and that of the liver (bile) are alkaline, as are also the blood and most juices of the body. The stomach juice is acid, as also are the urine and the perspiration.

[3] It is wonderfully elastic and constantly changing in size, contracting till it will scarcely hold a quart when empty, and expanding, as food or drink is put into it, until it will easily hold two quarts, or even a gallon or more when greatly distended, as by gas.

[4] If you take some pepsin which has been extracted from the stomach of a pig or a calf, melt it in water in a glass tube, then drop one or two little pieces of meat or hard-boiled white of egg into it, you can see them slowly melt

away like sugar in a cup of coffee. If you add a few drops of hydrochloric acid, the melting will go on much faster; and if you warm up the tube to about the heat of the body, it will proceed faster still. So nature knew just what she was doing when she provided pepsin and acid and warmth in the stomach.

[5] The liver and the bile are more fully described in chapter XVII.

[6] Tiny plant cells, known also as germs, which cause fermentation, decay, and many diseases.

CHAPTER III

THE FOOD-FUEL OF THE BODY-ENGINE

WHAT KIND OF FOOD SHOULD WE EAT?

Generally speaking, our Appetites will Guide us. Our whole body is an ingenious machine for catching food, digesting it, and turning the energy, or fuel value, which it contains, into life, movement, and growth.

Naturally, two things follow: first, that the kind and amount of food which we eat is of great importance; and second, that from the millions of years of experience that the human body has had in trying all sorts of foods, it has adapted itself to certain kinds of food and developed certain likes and dislikes which we call appetites. Those who happened to like unhealthy and unwholesome foods were poisoned, or grew thin and weak and died off, so that we are descended solely from people who had sound and reliable food appetites; and, in the main, what our instincts and appetites tell us about food is to be depended upon.

The main questions which we have to consider are: How much of the different kinds of food it is best for us to eat, and in what proportions we should use them. Both men and animals, since the world began, have been trying to eat and digest almost everything that they could get into their mouths. And what we now like and prepare as foods are the things which have stood the test, and proved themselves able to yield strength and nourishment to the body. So practically every food that comes upon our tables has some kind of real food value, or it wouldn't appear there.

The most careful study and analysis have shown that almost every known food has some peculiar advantage, such as digestibility, or cheapness, or pleasant taste as flavoring for other more nutritious, but less interesting, foods. But some foods have much higher degrees of nutritiousness or digestibility or wholesomeness than others; so that our problem is to pick out from a number of foods that "taste good" to us, those which are the most nutritious, the most digestible, and the most wholesome, and to see that we get plenty of them. It is not that certain foods, or classes of food, are "good," and should be eaten to the exclusion of all others; nor that certain foods, or classes of food, are "bad," and should be excluded from our tables entirely; but that certain foods are more nutritious, or more wholesome, than others; and that it is best to see that we get plenty of the former before indulging our appetites upon the latter.

Beware of Tainted Food. The most dangerous fault that any food can have is that it shall be tainted, or spoiled, or smell bad. Spoiling, or tainting, means that the food has become infected by some germs of putrefaction, generally bacteria or moulds (see chapter XXVI). It is the poisons--called ptomaines, or toxins--produced by these germs which cause the serious disturbances in the stomach, and not either the amount or the kind of food itself. Even a regular "gorge" upon early apples or watermelon or cake or ice cream will not give you half so bad, nor so dangerous, colic as one little piece of tainted meat or fish or egg, or one cupful of dirty milk, or a single helping of cabbage or tomatoes that have begun to spoil, or of jam made out of spoiled berries or other fruit. This spoiling can be prevented by strict cleanliness in handling foods, especially milk, meat, and fruit; by keeping foods screened from dust and flies; and by keeping them cool with ice in summer time, thus checking the growth of these "spoiling" germs. The refrigerator in the kitchen prevents colic or diarrhea, ice in hot weather is one of the necessaries of life. Smell every piece of food to be eaten, in the kitchen before it is cooked, if possible; but if not, at the table avoid everything that has an unpleasant odor, or tastes queer, and you will avoid two-thirds of the colic, diarrhea, and bilious attacks which are so often supposed to be due to eating too much.

Variety in Food is Necessary. Man has always lived on, and apparently required, a great variety of foods, animal and vegetable--fish and flesh, nuts, fruit, grains, fat, sugar, and vegetables. Indeed, it was probably because man could live on anything and everything that he was able to survive in famines and to get so far ahead of all other sorts of animals.

We still need a great variety of different sorts of food in order to keep our health; so our tendency to become tired of a certain food, after we have had it over and over and over again, for breakfast, dinner, and supper, is a sound and healthy one. There is no "best food"; nor is there any one food on which we can live and work, as an engine will work all its "life" on one kind of coal, wood, or oil. No one kind of food contains all the stuffs that our body is made of and needs, in exactly the right proportions. It takes a dozen or more different kinds of food to supply these, and the body picks out what it wants, and throws away the remainder.

Even the best and most nutritious and digestible single food, like meat, or bread and butter, or sugar, is not sufficient by itself; nor will it do for every meal in the day, or every day in the week. We must eat other things with it; and we must from time to time change it for something which may even be not quite so nutritious, in order to give our body the opportunity to select from a great variety of foods the particular things which its wonderful instincts and skill can use to build it up and keep it healthy. This is why every grocery store, every butcher shop, every fish market, and every confectioner's shows such a great variety of different kinds of foods put up and prepared in all sorts of ways. Although nearly two-thirds of the actual fuel which we put into our body-boilers is in the form of a dozen or fifteen great staple foods, like bread, meat, butter, sugar, eggs, milk, potatoes, and fish, yet all the lighter foods, also, are needed for perfect health.

It is possible, by careful selection, and by taking a great deal of trouble, to supply all the elements of the body from animal foods alone, or from vegetable foods alone. But practically, it has everywhere, and in all ages, been found that the best and most healthful diet is a proper combination of animal and vegetable foods. Our starches, for instance, which furnish most of our fuel,--though they give us comparatively little to build up, or repair, the body with,--are found, as we have seen, in the vegetable kingdom, in grains and fruits; while most of our proteins and fats, which chiefly give us the materials with which to build up, or repair, the body, are found in the animal kingdom. There is no advantage whatever in trying to exclude either animal food or vegetable food from our dietary. Both animal and vegetable foods are wholesome in their proper place, and their proper place is on the table together.

Those nations which live solely, or even chiefly, upon one or two kinds of staple foods, such as rice, potatoes, corn-meal, or yams, do so solely because they are too poor to afford other kinds of food, or too lazy, or too uncivilized, to get them; and instead of being healthier and longer-lived than civilized races, they are much more subject to disease and live only about half as long.

THE THREE GREAT CLASSES OF FOOD-FUEL

Food is Fuel. Now what is the chief quality which makes one kind of food preferable to another? As our body machine runs entirely upon the energy or "strength" which it gets out of its food, a good food must have plenty of fuel value; that is to say, it must be capable of burning and giving off heat and steaming-power. Other things being equal, the more it has of this fuel value, the more desirable and valuable it will be as a food.

From this point of view, foods may be roughly classified, after the fashion of the materials needed to build a fire in a grate or stove, as Coal foods, Kindling foods, and Paper foods. Although coal, kindling, and paper are of very different fuel values, they are all necessary to start the fire in the grate and to keep it burning properly. Moreover, any one of them would keep a fire going alone, after a fashion, provided that you had a grate or furnace large enough to burn it in, and could shovel it in fast enough; and the same is true, to a certain degree, of the foods in the body.

How to Judge the Fuel Value of Foods. One of the best ways of roughly determining whether a given food belongs in the Coal, the Kindling, or the Paper class, is to take a handful or spoonful of it, dry it thoroughly by some means,--evaporating, or driving off the water,--and then throw what is left into a fire and see how it will burn. A piece of beef, for instance, would shrink a good deal in drying; but about one-third of it would be left, and this dried beef would burn quite briskly and would last for some time in the fire. A piece of bread of the same size would not shrink so much, but would lose about the same proportion of its weight; and it also would burn with a clear, hot flame, though not quite so long as the beef. A piece of fat of the same size would shrink very little in drying and would burn with a bright, hot flame, nearly twice as long as either the beef or the bread. These would all be classed as Coal foods.

Then if we were to dry a slice of apple, it would shrink down into a little leathery shaving; and this, when thrown into the fire, would burn with a smudgy kind of flame, give off very little heat, and soon smoulder away. A piece of raw potato of the same size would shrink even more, but would give a hotter and cleaner flame. A leaf of cabbage, or a piece of beet-root, or four or five large strawberries would shrivel away in the drying almost to nothing and, if thoroughly dried, would disappear in a flash when thrown on the fire. These, then, except the potato, we should regard as Kindling foods.

But it would take a large handful of lettuce leaves, or a big cup of beef-tea, or a good-sized bowl of soup, or a big cucumber, or a gallon of tea or coffee, to leave sufficient solid remains when completely dried, to make more than a flash when thrown into the fire. These, then, are Paper foods, with little fuel value.

CHAPTER IV

THE COAL FOODS

Kinds of Coal Foods. There are many different kinds of Coal foods, such as pork, mutton, beef, bread, corn-cakes, bacon, potatoes, rice, sugar, cheese, butter, and so on. But when you come to look at them more closely, and to take them to pieces, or, as we say, analyze them, you will see that they all fall into three different kinds or classes: (1) Proteins, such as meat, milk, fish, eggs, cheese, etc. (2) Starch-sugars (carbohydrates), found pure as laundry starch and as white sugar; also found, as starch, making up the bulk of wheat and other grains, and of potatoes, rice, peas; also found, as sugar, in honey, beet-roots, sugar cane, and the sap of maple trees. (3) Fats, found in fat meats, butter, oil, nuts, beeswax, etc.

This whole class of Coal foods can be recognized by the fact that usually some one of them will form the staple, or main dish, of almost any regular meal, which is generally a combination of all three classes--a protein in the shape of meat; a starch-sugar in the form of bread, potatoes, or rice; and a fat in the form of butter in northern climates, or of olive oil in the tropics.

PROTEINS, OR "MEATS"

Proteins, the "First Foods." There are proteins, or "meats," both animal and vegetable; and no one can support life without protein in some form. This is because proteins alone contain sufficient amounts of the great element called nitrogen, which forms a large part of every portion of our bodies. This is why they are called proteins, meaning "first foods," or most necessary foods. Whatever we may live on in later life, we all began on a diet of liquid meat (milk), and could have survived and grown up on nothing else.

Composition of Proteins. Nearly all our meats are the muscle of different sorts of animals, made of a soft, reddish, animal pulp called myosin; the other principal proteins being white of egg, curd of milk, and a gummy, whitish-gray substance called gluten, found in wheat flour. This gluten is the stuff that makes the paste and dough of wheat flour sticky, so that you can paste things together with it; while that made from corn meal or oatmeal will fall to pieces when you take it up. The jelly-like or pulp-like myosin in meat is held together by strings or threads of tough, fibrous stuff; and the more there is of this fibrous material in a particular piece or "cut," of meat, the tougher and less juicy it is. The thick, soft muscles, which lie close under the backbone in the small of the back, in all animals, have less of this tough and indigestible fibrous stuff in them, and cuts across them give us the well-known porter-house, sirloin, or tenderloin steaks, and the best and tenderest mutton and pork chops.

Fuel Value of Meats. Weight for weight, most of the butcher's meats--beef, pork, mutton, and veal--have about the same food value, differing chiefly in the amount of fat that is mixed in with their fibres, and in certain flavoring substances, which give them, when roasted, or broiled, their special flavors. The different flavors are not of any practical importance, except in the case of mutton, which some people dislike and therefore can take only occasionally, and in small amounts.

The amount of fat in meats, however, is more important; and depends largely upon how well the animal has been fed. There is usually the least amount of fat in mutton, more in beef, and by far the greatest amount in pork. This fat adds to the fuel value of meat, but makes it a little slower of digestion; and its presence in large amounts in pork, together with the fact that it lies, not only in layers and streaks, but also mixed in between the fibres of the lean as well has caused this meat to be regarded as richer and more difficult of digestion than either beef or mutton. This, however is not quite fair to the pork, because smaller amounts of it will satisfy the appetite and furnish the body with sufficient fuel and nutrition. If it be eaten in moderate amounts and thoroughly chewed, it is a wholesome and valuable food.

Veal is slightly less digestible than beef or mutton, on account of the amount of slippery gelatin in and among its fibres; but if well cooked and well chewed, it is wholesome.

The other meats--chicken, duck, and other poultry, game, etc.--are of much less nutritive value than either beef, pork, or mutton, partly because of the large amount of waste in them, in the form of bones, skin, and tendons, and partly from the greater amount of water in them. But their flavors make them an agreeable change from the staple meats.

Fish belongs in the same class as poultry and consists of the same muscle substance, but, as you can readily see by the way that it shrinks when dried, contains far more water and has less fuel value. Some of the richer and more solid fishes, like salmon, halibut, and mackerel, contain, in addition to their protein, considerable amounts of fat and, when dried or cured, give a rather high fuel value at moderate cost. But the peculiar flavor of fish, its large percentage of water, and the special make-up of its protein, give it a very low food value, and render it, on the whole, undesirable as a permanent staple food. Races and classes who live on it as their chief meat-food are not so vigorous or so healthy as those who eat also the flesh of animals. As a rule, it is not best to use fish as the main dish of a meal oftener than two or three times a week.

Milk. Milk is an interesting food of great value because it combines in itself all three of the great classes of food-stuffs,--protein, starch-sugar, and fat. Its protein is a substance called casein, which forms the bulk of curds, and which, when dried and salted, is called cheese. The fat is present in little tiny globules which give milk its whitish or milky color. When milk is allowed to stand, these globules of fat, being lighter, float up to the top and form a layer which is called cream. When this cream is skimmed off and put into a churn, and shaken or beaten violently so as to break the little film with which each of these droplets is coated, they run together and form a yellow mass which we call butter. In addition to the curd and fat, milk contains also sugar, called milk-sugar (lactose), which gives it its sweetish taste. And as a considerable part of the casein, or curd, is composed of another starch-like body, or animal starch, this makes milk quite rich in the starch-sugar group of food-stuffs.

All these substances, of course, in milk are dissolved in a large amount of water, so that when milk is evaporated, or dried, it shrinks down to barely one-sixth of its former bulk. It is, in fact, a liquid meat, starch-sugar, and fat in one; and that is why babies are able to live and thrive on it alone for the first six months of their lives. It is also a very valuable food for older children, though, naturally, it is not "strong" enough and needs to be combined with bread, puddings, meat, and fat.

Soups and Broths. Soups, broths, and beef teas are water in which meats, bones, and other scraps have been boiled. They are about ninety-eight per cent water, and contain nothing of the meat or bones except some of their flavor, and a little gelatin. They have little or no nutritive or fuel value, and are really Paper foods, useful solely as stimulants to appetite and digestion, enabling us to swallow with relish large pieces of bread or crackers, or the potatoes, rice, pea-meal, cheese, or other real foods with which they are thickened. Their food value has been greatly exaggerated, and many an unfortunate invalid has literally starved on them. Ninety-five per cent of the food value of the meat and bones, out of which soups are made, remains at the bottom of the pot, after the soup has been poured off. The commercial extracts of meat are little better than frauds, for they contain practically nothing but flavoring matters.

Protein in Vegetables. Several vegetable substances contain considerable amounts of protein. One of these has already been mentioned,--the gluten or sticky part of bread,--and this is what has given wheat its well-deserved reputation as the best of all grains out of which to make flour for human food.

There is also another vegetable protein, called legumin, found in quite large amounts in dried beans and peas; but this is of limited food value, first because it is difficult of digestion, and secondly because with it, in dried peas and beans, are found a pungent oil and a bitter substance, which give them their peculiar strong flavor, both of which are quite irritating to the average person's digestion. So distressing and disturbing are these flavoring substances to the civilized stomach, that, after thousands of attempts to use them more largely, it has been found that a full meal of beans once or twice a week is all that the comfort and health of the body will stand. This is really a great pity, for beans and peas are both nourishing and cheap. Nuts also contain much protein, but are both difficult of digestion and expensive.

Virtues and Drawbacks of Meats. Taken all together, the proteins, or meats, are the most nutritious and wholesome single class of foods. Their chief drawback is their expense, which, in proportion to their fuel value, is greater than that of the starches. Then, on account of their attractiveness, they may be eaten at times in too large amounts. They are also somewhat more difficult to keep and preserve than are either the starches or the fats. The old idea that, when burned up in the body, they give rise to waste products, which are either more poisonous or more difficult to get rid of than those of vegetable foods, is now regarded as having no sufficient foundation. Neither is the common belief that meats cause gout well founded.

The greatest danger connected with meats is that they may become tainted, or begin to spoil, or decay, before they are used. Unfortunately, the ingenious cook has invented a great many ways of smothering, or disguising, the well-marked bad taste of decayed, or spoiled, meat by spices, onions, and savory herbs. So, as a general thing, the safest plan, especially when traveling or living away from home, is to avoid as far as possible hashes, stews, and other "made" dishes containing meat. This is one of the ways in which spices and onions have got such a bad reputation for "heating the blood," or upsetting the stomach, when it is really the decayed meat which they are used to disguise that causes the trouble. Highly spiced dishes rob you of the services of your best guide to the wholesomeness of food--your nose.

Risks of Dirty Milk. The risks from tainting or spoiling are particularly great in the case of milk, partly on account of the dusty and otherwise uncleanly barns and sheds in which it is often handled and kept, and from which it is loaded with a heavy crop of bacteria at the very start; and partly because the same delicateness which makes it so easily digestible for babies, makes it equally easy for germs and bacteria to grow in it and spoil, or sour, it. You all know how disagreeable the taste of spoiled milk is; and it is as dangerous as it is disagreeable. A very large share of the illnesses of babies and young children, particularly the diseases of stomach and bowels which are so common in hot weather, are due to the use of spoiled, dirty milk.

There is one sure preventive for all these dangers, and that is absolute cleanliness from cow to customer. All the changes that take place in milk are caused by germs of various sorts, usually floating in the air, that get into it. If the milk is so handled and protected, from cow to breakfast table, that these germs cannot get into it, it will remain sweet for several days.

Boards of Health all over the world now are insisting upon absolutely clean barns and cleanly methods of handling, shipping, and selling milk. In most of our large cities, milk-men are not allowed to sell milk without a license; and this license is granted only after a thorough examination of their cattle, barns, and milk-houses. These clean methods of handling milk cost very little; they take only time and pains.

Nowadays, in the best dairies, it is required that the barns or sheds in which cows are milked shall have tight walls and roofs and good flooring; that the walls and roofs shall be kept white-washed; and the floor be cleaned and washed before each milking, so that no germs from dust or manure can float into the milk. Then the cows are kept in a clean pasture, or dry, graveled yard, instead of a muddy barnyard; and are either brushed, or washed down with a hose before each milking, so that no dust or dirt will fall from them into the milk. The men who are to milk wash their hands thoroughly with soap and water, and put on clean white canvas or cotton overalls, jackets, and caps. As soon as the milk has been drawn into the pails, it is carried into the milk-room and cooled down to a temperature of about forty-two degrees--that is, about ten degrees above freezing point. This is to prevent the growth of such few germs as may have got into it, in spite of all the care that has been taken. Then the milk is drawn into bottles; and the bottles are tightly capped by a water-proof pasteboard disc, or cover, which is not removed until the milk is brought into the house and poured into the glass, or cup, for use.

Milk handled like this costs from two to four cents a quart more to produce than when drawn from a cow smeared with manure, in a dark, dirty, strong-smelling barn, by a milker with greasy clothing and dirty hands; and then ladled out into pitchers in the open street, giving all the dust and flies that happen to be in the neighborhood a chance to get into it! But it is doubly worth the extra price, because, besides escaping stomach and bowel troubles, you get more cream and higher food value. There is one-third more food value in clean milk than in dirty milk, because its casein and sugar have not been spoiled and eaten by swarms of bacteria. How great a difference careful cleanliness of this sort can make in milk is shown by the difference in the number of bacteria that the two kinds of milk contain. Ordinary milk bought from the wagons in the open street, or from the cans in the stores, will contain anywhere from a million to a million and a half bacteria to the cubic centimeter (about fifteen drops); and samples have actually been taken and counted, which showed five and six millions.

Such a splendid food for germs is milk, and so rapidly do they grow in it, that dirty milk will actually contain more of them to the cubic inch than sewage, as it flows in the sewers. Now see what a difference a little cleanliness will make! Good, clean, carefully handled milk, instead of having a million, or a million and a half, bacteria, will have less than ten thousand; and very clean milk may contain as low as three or four hundred, and these of harmless sorts. The whole gospel of the care of milk can be summed up in two sentences: (1) Keep dirt and germs out of the milk. (2) Keep the milk cool.

Besides the germs of the summer diseases of children, which kill more than fifty thousand babies every year in the United States, dirty milk may also contain typhoid germs and consumption germs. The typhoid germs do not come from the body of the cow, but get into the milk through its being handled by people who have, or have just recovered from, typhoid, or who are nursing patients sick with typhoid, and who have not properly washed their hands; or from washing the cans, or from watering the milk with water taken from a well or stream infected with typhoid. It is estimated that about one-eighth of all the half million cases of typhoid that occur in the United States every year are carried through dirty milk.

The germs of consumption, or tuberculosis, that are present in milk may come from a cow that has the disease; or from consumptive human beings who handle the milk; or from the dust of streets or houses--which often contains disease germs. The latter sources are far the more dangerous; for, as is now pretty generally agreed, although the tuberculosis of cattle can be given to human beings, it is not very actively dangerous to them; and probably not more than three or four per cent of all cases of tuberculosis come from this source. The idea, however, of allowing the milk of cows diseased from any cause to be used for human food, is not to be tolerated for a moment. All good dairymen and energetic Boards of Health now insist upon dairy herds being tested for tuberculosis, and the killing, or weeding out, of all cows that show they have the disease.

Cheese. Cheese is the curd of milk squeezed dry of its liquid (whey), salted, pressed into a mould, and allowed to ferment slowly, or "ripen," in which process a considerable part of its casein is turned into fat. It is a cheap, concentrated, and very nutritious food, and in small amounts is quite appetizing. But unfortunately, the acids and extracts which have formed in the process of fermentation and ripening are so irritating to the stomach, that it can usually be eaten only in small amounts, without upsetting the digestion. Its chief value is as a relish with bread, crackers, potatoes, or macaroni. In moderate amounts, it is not only appetizing and digestible, but will assist in the digestion of other foods; hence the custom of eating a small piece of "ripe" cheese at the end of a heavy meal.

CHAPTER V

THE COAL FOODS (Continued)

STARCHES

Sources of Starch. The starches are valuable and wholesome foods. They form the largest part, both in bulk and in fuel value, of our diet, and have done so ever since man learned how to cultivate the soil and grow crops of grain. The reason is clear: One acre of good land will grow from ten to fifteen times the amount of food in the form of starch in grains or roots, as of meat in the shape of cattle or sheep. Consequently, starch is far cheaper, and this is its great advantage.

Our chief supply of starch is obtained from the seed of certain most useful grasses, which we call wheat, oats, barley, rye, rice, and corn, and from the so-called "roots" of the potato. Potatoes are really underground buds packed with starch, and their proper name is tubers.

Starch, when pure or extracted, is a soft, white powder, which you have often seen as cornstarch, or laundry starch. As found in grains, it is mixed with a certain amount of vegetable fibre, covered with husks, or skin, and has the little germ or budlet of the coming plant inside it. It has been manufactured and laid down by little cells inside their own bodies, which make up the grains; so that each particular grain of starch is surrounded by a delicate husk--the wall of the cell that made it. This means that grains and other starch foods have to be prepared for eating by grinding and cooking. The grinding crushes the grains into a powder so that the starch can be sifted out from the husks and coating of the grain, and the fibres which hold it together; and the cooking causes the tiny starch grain to swell and burst the cell wall, or bag, which surrounds it.

Starches as Fuel. The starches contain no nitrogen except a mere trace in the framework of the grains or roots they grow in. They burn very clean; that is, almost the whole of them is turned into carbon dioxid gas and water.[7]

This burning quality makes the starches a capital fuel both in the body and out of it. You may have heard of how settlers out on the prairies, who were a long way from a railroad and had no wood or coal, but plenty of corn, would fill their coal scuttles with corn and burn that in their stoves; and a very bright, hot fire it made.

One of the chief weaknesses of the starches is that they burn up too fast, so that you get hungry again much more quickly after a meal made entirely upon starchy foods, like bread, crackers, potatoes, or rice, than you do after one which has contained some meat, particularly fat, which burns and digests more slowly.

How Starch is Changed into Sugar. As we learned in chapter II, the starches can be digested only after they are turned into sugars in the body. If you put salt with sugar or starch, although it will mix perfectly and give its taste to the mixture, neither the salt nor the starch nor the sugar will have changed at all, but will remain exactly as it was in the first place, except for being mixed with the other substances. But if you were to pour water containing an acid over the starch, and then boil it for a little time, your starch would entirely disappear, and something quite different take its place. This, when you tasted it, you would find was sweet; and, when the water was boiled off, it would turn out to be a sugar called glucose. Again, if you should pour a strong acid over sawdust, it would "char" it, or change it into another substance, carbon. In both of these cases--that of the starch and of the sawdust--what we call a chemical change would have taken place between the acid and the starch, and between the strong acid and the sawdust.

If we looked into the matter more closely, we should find that what has happened is that the starch and the sawdust have changed into quite different substances. Starches are insoluble in water; that is, although they can be softened and changed into a jelly-like substance, they cannot be completely melted, or dissolved, like salt or sugar. Sugar, on the other hand, is a perfectly soluble or "meltable" substance, and can soak or penetrate through any membrane or substance in the body. Therefore all the starches which we eat--bread, biscuit, potato, etc.--have to be acted upon by the ferments of our saliva and our pancreatic juice, and turned into sugar, called glucose, which can be easily poured into the blood and carried wherever it is needed, all over the body. Thus we see what a close relation there is between starch and sugar, and why the group we are studying is sometimes called the starch-sugars.

Wheat--our Most Valuable Starch Food. The principal forms in which starch comes upon our tables are meals and flours, and the various breads, cakes, mushes, and puddings made out of these. Far the most valuable and important of all is wheat flour, because this grain contains, as we have seen, not only starch, but a considerable amount of vegetable "meat," or gluten, which is easily digested in the stomach. This gluten, however, carries with it one disadvantage--its stickiness, or gumminess. The dough or paste made by mixing wheat flour with water is heavy and wet, or, as we say, "soggy," as compared with that made by mixing oatmeal or corn meal or rice flour with water. If it is baked in this form, it makes a well-flavored, but rather tough, leathery sort of crust; so those races that use no leavening, or rising-stuff, in their wheat bread, roll it out into very thin sheets and bake it on griddles or hot stones.

Most races that have wheat, however, have hit upon a plan for overcoming this heaviness and sogginess, and that is the rather ingenious one of mixing some substance in the dough which will give off bubbles of a gas, carbon dioxid, and cause it to puff up and become spongy and light, or, as we say, "full of air." This is what gives bread its well-known spongy or porous texture; but the tiny cells and holes in it are filled, not with air, but with carbon dioxid gas.

Making Bread with Yeast. There are several ways of lightening bread with carbon dioxid gas. The oldest and commonest is by mixing in with the flour and water a small amount of the frothy mass made by a germ, or microbe, known as yeast or the yeast plant. Then the dough is set away in a warm place "to rise," which means that the busy little yeast cells, eagerly attacking the rich supply of starchy food spread before them, and encouraged by the heat and moisture, multiply by millions and billions, and in the process of growing and multiplying, give off, like all other living cells, the gas, carbon dioxid. This bubbles and spreads all through the mass, the dough begins to rise, and finally swells right above the pan or crock in which it was set. If it is allowed to stand and rise too long, it becomes sour, because the yeast plant is forming, at the same time, three other substances--alcohol, lactic acid (which gives an acid taste to the bread), and vinegar. Usually they form in such trifling amounts as to be quite unnoticeable. When the bread has become light enough, it is put into the oven to be baked.

The baking serves the double purpose of cooking and thus making the starch appetizing, and of killing the yeast germs so that they will carry their fermentation no further. Bread that has not been thoroughly baked, if it is kept too long, will turn sour, because some of the yeast germs that have escaped will set to work again.

That part of the dough that lies on the surface of the loaf, and is exposed to the direct heat of the oven has its starch changed into a substance somewhat like sugar, known as dextrin, which, with the slight burning of the carbon, gives the outside, or crust, of bread its brownish color, its crispness, and its delicious taste. The crust is really the most nourishing part of the loaf, as well as the part that gives best exercise to the teeth.

Making Bread with Soda or Baking-Powders. Another method of giving lightness to bread is by mixing an acid like sour milk and an alkali like soda with the flour, and letting them effervesce[8] and give off carbon dioxid. This is the mixture used in making the famous "soda biscuit." Still another method is by the use of baking-powders, which are made of a mixture of some cheap and harmless acid powder with an alkaline powder--usually some form of soda. As long as these powders are kept dry, they will not act upon each other; but as soon as they are moistened in the dough, they begin to give off carbon dioxid gas.

Neither sour milk and soda nor baking-powder will make as thoroughly light and spongy and digestible bread as will yeast. If, however, baking-powders are made of pure and harmless materials, used in proper proportions so as just to neutralize each other, and thus leave no excess of acid or alkali, and if the bread is baked very thoroughly, they make a wholesome and nutritious bread, which has the advantage of being very quickly and easily made. The chief objection to soda or baking-powder bread is that, being often made in a hurry, the acid and the alkali do not get thoroughly mixed all through the flour, and consequently do not raise or lighten the dough properly, and the loaf or biscuit is likely to be heavy and soggy in the centre. This heavy, soggy stuff can be neither properly chewed in the mouth, nor mixed with the digestive juices, and hence is difficult to digest. If, however, soda biscuits are made thin and baked thoroughly so as to make them at least half or two-thirds crust, they are perfectly digestible and wholesome, and furnish a valuable and appetizing variety for our breakfast and supper tables.

Bran or Brown Bread. Flour made by grinding the wheat-berry without sifting the husks, or bran, out of it is called "whole-wheat" meal; and bread made from it is the brown "bran bread" or "Graham bread." It was at one time supposed that because brown bread contained more nitrogen than white bread, it was more wholesome and nutritious, but this has been found to be a mistake, because the extra nitrogen in the brown bread is in the form of husks and fibres, which the stomach is quite unable to digest. Weight for weight, white bread is more nutritious than brown. The husks and fibres, however, which will not digest, pass on through the bowels unchanged and stir up the walls of the intestines to contract; hence they are useful in small quantities in helping to keep the bowels regular. But, like any other stimulus, too much of it will irritate and disturb the digestion, and cause diarrhea; so that it is not best to eat more than one-fifth of our total bread in the form of brown bread. Dyspeptics who live on brown bread, or on so-called "health foods," are simply feeding their dyspepsia.

"Breakfast Foods." The same defect exists in most of the breakfast cereals which flood our tables and decorate our bill-boards. Some of these are made of the waste of flouring mills, known as "middlings," "shorts," or bran, which were formerly used for cow-feed. The claims of many of them are greatly exaggerated, for they contain no more nourishment, or in no more digestible form, than the same weight of bread; and they cost from two to five times as much. As they come on our tables, they are nearly seven-eighths water; and the cream and sugar taken with them are of higher food value than they are. They should never be relied upon as the main part of a meal.

Corn Meal. Corn meal is one of the richest meals in nutritive value for its price, as it has an abundance of starch and a small amount of fat. It is, however, poor in nitrogen, and like the other grains, in countries where wheat will grow, it is chiefly valuable for furnishing cakes, fritters, and mushes to give variety to the diet, and help to regulate the bowels.

Oatmeal. Oatmeal comes the nearest to wheat in the amount of nitrogen or protein, but the digestible part of this is much smaller than in wheat, and the indigestible portion is decidedly irritating to the bowels, so that if used in excess of about one-fifth of our total starch-food required, it is likely to upset the digestion.

Rye. Rye also contains a considerable amount of gluten, but is much poorer in starch than wheat is; and the bread made out of its flour--the so-called "black bread" of France and Germany--is dark, sticky, and inclined to sour readily. Most of the "rye" bread sold in the shops, or served on our tables, is made of wheat flour with a moderate mixture of rye to give the sour taste.

Rice. Rice consists chiefly of starch, and makes nutritious puddings or cakes, and may be used as a vegetable, in the place of potatoes, with meat and fish. It is, however, lacking in flavor, and when properly cooked, contains so much water that it has to be eaten in very large amounts to furnish much nutrition.

Potatoes. The only important starchy food outside of the grains is potatoes. These contain considerable amounts of starch, but mixed with a good deal of cellulose, or vegetable fibre, and water, so that, like rice, large amounts of them must be eaten in order to furnish a good fuel supply. They, however, make a very necessary article of diet in connection with meats, fish, and other vegetables.

As a rough illustration of the fuel value of the different starch foods, it may be said that in order to get the amount of nourishment contained in an ordinary pound loaf of wheat or white bread, it would be necessary to eat about seven pounds of cooked rice, as it comes on the table; about twelve pounds of boiled potatoes; or a bowl of oatmeal porridge about the size of a wash-basin.

SUGARS

Where Sugar is Obtained. The other great member of the starch, or carbohydrate, group of foods is sugar. This is a scarcer and more expensive food than starch because, instead of being found in solid masses in grains and roots like starch, it is scattered, very thinly, through the fruits, stems, and roots of a hundred different plants, seldom being present in greater amounts than two or three per cent. It is, however, so valuable a food, with so high a fuel value, and is so rapidly digested and absorbed, that man has always had a very keen desire for it, or, as we say, a "sweet tooth," and has literally searched the whole vegetable kingdom the world over to discover plants from which it could be secured in larger amounts. During the last two hundred years it has been obtained chiefly from two great sources: the juicy stem of a tall, coarse reed, or cane, the sugar-cane, growing in the tropics; and (within the last fifty years) the sweet juice of the large root of a turnip-like plant, the beet. Another source of sugar, in the earlier days of this country, was the juice or sap of the sugar maple, which is still greatly relished as a luxury, chiefly in the form of syrup.

Honey is nearly pure sugar together with certain ferments and flavoring extracts, derived in part from the flowers from which it is gathered, and in part from the stomach, or crop, of the bee.

The Food Value of Sugar. In the early days of its use, sugar, on account of its expensiveness, was looked upon solely as a luxury, and used sparingly--either as a flavoring for less attractive foods, or as a special treat; and like most new foods, it was declared to be unwholesome and dangerous. But sugar is now recognized as one of our most useful and valuable foods. In fuel value, it is the equal, indeed the superior, weight for weight, of starch; and as all starch has to be changed into it before it can be used by the body, it is evident that sugar is more easily digested and absorbed than starch, and furnishes practically a ready-made fuel for our muscles.

How We should Use Sugar. The drawbacks of sugar are that, on account of its exceedingly attractive taste, we may eat too much of it; and that, because it is so satisfying, if we do eat too much of it either between meals or at the beginning of meals, our appetites will be "killed" before we have really eaten a sufficient supply of nourishing food. But all we have to do to avoid these dangers is to use common sense and a little self-control, without which any one of our appetites may lead us into trouble.

On account of this satisfying property, sugar is best eaten at, or near, the close of a meal; and taken at that time, there is no objection to its use nearly pure, as in the form of sweet-meats, or good wholesome candy. Its alleged injurious effects upon the teeth are largely imaginary and no greater than those of the starchy foods. The teeth of various tropical races which live almost entirely on sugar-cane during certain seasons of the year are among the finest in the world; and any danger may be entirely avoided by proper brushing and cleaning of the teeth and gums after eating.

If eaten in excess, sugar quickly gives rise to fermentation in the stomach and bowels; but so do the starches and the fats, if over-indulged in. Its real value as a food may be judged from the fact that the German army has made it a part of its field ration in the shape of cakes of chocolate, and that the United States Government buys pure candy by the ton, for the use of its soldiers.

FOOTNOTES:

[7] On this account, they are often spoken of as carbohydrates, or "carbon-water stuffs."

[8] See page 11.

CHAPTER VI

THE COAL FOODS (Continued)

ANIMAL FATS

The Digestibility of Fats. We have now come to the last group of the real Coal foods, namely, the fats. Fats are the "hottest" and most concentrated fuel that we possess, and might be described as the "anthracites," or "hard coals" of our Coal foods. They are, also, as might be expected from their "strength" or concentration, among the slowest to digest of all our foods, so that, as a rule, we can eat them only in very moderate amounts, seldom exceeding one-tenth to one-sixth of our total food-fuel. It is not, however, quite correct to say that fats are hard to digest, because, although from their solid, oily character, they take a longer time to become digested and absorbed by the body than most other foods, yet they are as perfectly and as completely digested, with the healthy person, as any other kind of food. Indeed, it is this slowness of digestion which gives them their well-known staying-power as a food.

Their Place in our Diet. The wholesomeness of fats is well shown by our appetite for them, which is very keen for small amounts of them--witness, for instance, how quickly we notice and how keenly we object to the absence of butter on our bread or potatoes. To have our "bread well-buttered" is a well known expression for comfort and good fortune; yet a very little excess will turn our enjoyment into disgust. Fat, and particularly the cold fat of meat, "gags" us if we try to eat too much of it.

Fortunately, most of these fat-foods are quite expensive, pound for pound, and hence we are not often tempted to eat them in excess. Within proper limits, then, fats are an exceedingly important and useful food--a valuable member of the great family of Coal foods.

The Advantages of Fat as a Ration. The high fuel value and the small bulk of fats give them a very great practical advantage whenever supplies of food have to be carried for long distances, or for considerable lengths of time, as in sea voyages and hunting and exploring trips. So that in provisioning ships for a long voyage, or fitting out an expedition for the Arctic regions, fats, in the shape of bacon or pork, pemmican,[9] or the richer dried fishes, like salmon, mackerel, and herring, will be found to play an important part. Fats also have the great advantage, like the starches, of keeping well for long periods, especially after they have been melted and sterilized by boiling, or "rendering," as in the case of lard, or have had moderate amounts of salt added to them, as in butter.

If you were obliged to pick out a ration which would keep you alive, give you working power, and fit into the smallest possible bulk, you would take a protein, a sugar, and a fat in about equal amounts. Indeed, the German emergency field-ration, intended to keep soldiers in the field for three or four days without their baggage-wagons, or cook-trains, is made up of bacon, pea-meal, and chocolate. A small packet of these, which weighs only a little over two pounds, and which can be slipped into the knapsack, will, with plenty of water, keep a soldier in fighting trim for three days.

Butter. The most useful and wholesome single fat is the one which is in greatest demand--butter. This, as we have seen, is the churned and concentrated fat of milk, to which a little salt has been added to keep the milk-acid (lactic acid) which cannot be entirely washed out of it, from "turning it sour" or rancid. The rancid, offensive taste of bad or "strong" butter is due to the formation of another acid call butyric ("buttery") acid.

Butter is the best and most wholesome of our common fats because it is most easily digested, most readily absorbed, and least likely to give rise to this butyric acid fermentation. We should be particularly careful, even more so almost than with other foods, to see that it is perfectly sweet and good, because when we swallow rancid butter, we are simply swallowing a ready-made attack of indigestion. Most people's stomachs are strong enough to deal with small amounts of rancid butter without discomfort; but it is a strain on them that ought to be avoided, especially when good butter is simply a matter of strict cleanliness and care in handling and churning the cream, and of keeping the butter cool after it has been made.

Plenty of sweet butter is one of the most important and necessary elements in our diet, especially in childhood. And if children are allowed to eat pretty nearly as much as they want of it on their bread or potatoes, and plenty of its liquid form, cream, on their berries and puddings, it will save the necessity of many a dose of cod-liver oil, or bitter physic. Cream is far superior to either cod-liver or castor oil for keeping us in health.

Oleomargarine. On account of the expensiveness of butter, there are a number of substitutes sold, which go under the name of oleomargarine. These are made of the fat, or suet, of beef or mutton, mixed with a certain amount of cream and real butter, to give them an agreeable flavor. They are wholesome and useful fats, and for cooking purposes may very largely be substituted for butter. Owing to the fact that their fat is freer from the milk acids, they keep better than butter; and sweet, sound oleomargarine is to be preferred to rank, rancid butter. But it is not so readily digestible as butter is; is more liable to give rise to the butyric acid fermentations in the stomach; is not nearly so appetizing; and its sale as, and under the name of, butter is a fraud which the law rightly forbids and punishes.

Lard. The next most useful and generally used pure fat is lard--the rendered, or boiled-down, fat of pork. It is a useful substitute for butter in cooking, where butter is scarce. But, even in pastry or cakes, it has neither the flavor nor the digestibility of butter, and the latter should always be used when it can be had.

Bacon and Ham. The most useful and digestible fat meats are bacon and ham, as the dried, salted, and usually smoked, meat of the pig is called. Like all other fats, they can be eaten only in moderate amounts; but thus eaten, they are both appetizing, digestible, and very nutritious. One good slice of breakfast bacon, for instance, contains as much fuel value as two large saucers of mush or breakfast food, or two eggs, or two large slices of bread, or three oranges, or two small glasses of milk, or a quart of berries.

NUTS

How Nuts should be Used. Another form of fat is the "meat" of different nuts--walnuts, pecans, almonds, etc. These are quite rich in fats, and also contain a fair amount of proteins, and are, in small quantities, like other fats, appetizing and useful articles of food. But they should not be depended upon to furnish more than a small amount of the whole food supply, or even of its necessary fat, because nearly all nuts contain pungent or bitter aromatic oils and ferments, which give them their flavors, but which are likely to upset the digestion. This is particularly true of the peanut, which is not a true nut at all, but is, as its name indicates, a kind of pea grown underground. Peanuts, on account of their large amount of these irritating substances, are among the most indigestible and undesirable articles of diet in common use. A certain amount of these irritating substances present in nuts may be destroyed by careful roasting and salting; but this must be most carefully done, and it shrinks them in bulk so that the finished product is far more expensive than butter or fat meat of the same nutritive value. Good salted almonds, for instance, cost fifty to eighty cents a pound.

The proper place for nuts is where they usually come on our tables--at the end of a meal. Those who attempt to cure themselves of dyspepsia by a nut diet are simply making permanent their disease.

FOOTNOTES:

[9] Pemmican is a sort of "canned beef" made originally out of the best parts of venison and buffalo-meat. This is boiled, and packed into skin bags; then melted fat is poured in, so as to fill up all the chinks and form a thick layer over the surface. It is now made of beef packed in canvas bags, and is much used by polar expeditions and Alaskan miners.

CHAPTER VII

KINDLING AND PAPER FOODS--FRUITS AND VEGETABLES

The Special Uses of Fruits and Vegetables. We come now to the very much larger but much less important class of foods--the Kindling foods, which help the Coal foods to burn, and supply certain stuffs and elements which the body needs and which the coal foods do not contain. These are the vegetables--other than potatoes and dried peas and beans--and fruits.

Fruits and vegetables contain certain mineral elements, which are not present in sufficient proportions in the meats, starches, and fats. Furthermore, the products of their digestion and burning in the body help to neutralize, or render harmless, the waste products from meats, starches, and fats. Thirdly, they have a very beneficial effect upon the blood, the kidneys, and the skin. In fact, the reputation of fruits and fresh vegetables for "purifying the blood" and "clearing the complexion" is really well deserved. The keenness of our liking for fruit at all times, and our special longing for greens and sour things in the spring, after their scarcity in our diet all winter, is a true sign of their wholesomeness.

Not the least of their advantages is that they contain a very large proportion of water; and this, though diminishing their fuel value, supplies the body with a naturally filtered and often distilled supply of this necessary element of life. One of the best ways of avoiding that burning summer thirst, which leads you to flood your unfortunate stomach with melted icebergs, in the form of ice water, ice cold lemonade, or soda water, is to take an abundance of fresh fruits and green vegetables.

Many of the vegetables contain small amounts of starch, but few of them enough to count upon as fuel, except potatoes, which we have already classed with the Coal foods. Most fruits contain a certain amount of sugar-- how much can usually be estimated from their taste, and how little can be gathered from the statement that even the sweetest of fruits, like ripe pears or ripe peaches, contain only about eight per cent of sugar. They are all chiefly useful as flavors for the less interesting staple foods, particularly the starches. In fact, our instinctive use of them to help down bread and butter, or rice, or puddings of various sorts, is a natural and proper one. Like the vegetables, they contain various salts which are useful in neutralizing certain acid substances formed in the body. Soldiers in war, or sailors upon long voyages, who are fed upon a diet consisting chiefly of salted or preserved meat, with bread or hard biscuit and sugar, but without either fruits or fresh vegetables, are likely to develop a disease called scurvy. Little more than a century ago, hundreds of deaths occurred every year in the British and French navies from this disease, and the crews of many a long exploring voyage--like Captain Cook's--or of searchers for the North Pole, have been completely disabled or even destroyed entirely by scurvy. It was discovered that by adding to the diet fruit, or fresh vegetables like cabbage or potatoes, scurvy could be entirely prevented, or cured.[10]

Their Low Fuel Value. How little real fuel value fruits and vegetables have, may be easily seen from the following table. In order to get the nourishment contained in a pound loaf of bread, or a pound of roast beef, you would have to eat: 12 large apples or pears (5 lbs.); 4-1/2 qts. of strawberries; a dozen bananas (3-1/2 lbs.); 7 lbs. of onions; 2 doz. large cucumbers (18 lbs.); 10 lbs. of cabbage; 1/2 bushel of lettuce or celery.

Apples, the most Wholesome Fruit. Head and shoulders above all the other fruits stands that delight of our childhood days, apples. Well ripened, or properly cooked, they are readily digested by the average stomach; though some delicate digestions have difficulty with them. They contain a fair amount of acids, and from five to seven per cent of sugar. Their general wholesomeness and permanent usefulness may be gathered from the fact that they are one of the few fruits which you can eat almost daily the year round, or at very frequent intervals, without getting tired of them. Food that you don't get tired of is usually food which is good for you.

Dried apples are much inferior to the fresh fruit, because they become toughened in drying, and because growers sometimes smoke them with fumes of sulphur in the process, in order to bleach or whiten them; and this turns them into a sort of vegetable leather.

Other Fruits--their Advantages and Drawbacks. Next in usefulness probably come pears, though these have the disadvantage of containing a woody fibre, which is rather hard to digest, and they are, of course, poorer "keepers" than apples. Then come peaches, which have one of the most delicious flavors of all fruits, but which tend to set up fermentation and irritation in delicate stomachs, though in the average stomach, when eaten in moderation, they are wholesome and good. Then come the berries--strawberries, raspberries, blackberries,--all excellent and wholesome, when fresh in their season, or canned or preserved.

One warning, however, should be given about these most delicious, fragrant berries; and as it happens to apply also to several of our most attractive foods, it is well to mention it here. While perfectly wholesome and good for the majority of people, strawberries, for instance, are to a few--perhaps one in twenty--so irritating and indigestible as to be mildly poisonous. The other foods which may play this kind of trick with the stomachs of certain persons are oranges, bananas, melons, clams, lobsters, oysters, cheese, sage, and parsley, and occasionally, but very rarely, eggs and mutton. This is a matter which each of you can readily find out by experiment. If strawberries, melons, and other fruits agree with you, then eat freely of them, in due moderation. But if, after three or four trials, you find that they do not agree with you, but make your stomach burn, and perhaps give you an attack of nettle-rash or hives, or a headache, then let them alone.

The banana is of some food value because it contains not only sugar, but considerable quantities of starch--about the same amount as potatoes. But, if bananas are not fully ripe, both their starch and sugar are highly indigestible; while, if over-ripe, they have developed in them irritating substances, which are likely to upset the digestion and cause hives or eczema, especially in children. Bananas should therefore be regarded rather as a luxury and an agreeable variety than as a substantial part of the diet.

Food Values of the Different Vegetables. The vegetables depend for their value almost solely upon the alkaline salts and the water in them, and upon their flavor, which gives an agreeable variety to the diet. Parsnips, beets, and carrots are among the most nutritious, as they contain some starch and sugar; but they so quickly pall upon the taste that they can be used only in small amounts.

Turnips and cabbages possess the merit of being cheap and very easily grown. They contain valuable earthy salts, plenty of pure water, and a trace of starch. But these advantages are offset by their large amount of tough, woody vegetable fibre; this is incapable of digestion, and though in moderate amounts it is valuable in helping to regulate the movements of the bowels, in excess it soon becomes irritating. Both of them, particularly cabbages, contain, also, certain flavoring extracts, very rich in sulphur and exceedingly irritating to the stomach, which cause them to disagree with some persons. If these are got rid of by brisk boiling in at least two waters, then cabbage is a fairly wholesome and digestible dish for the average stomach. And because of its cheapness and "keeping" power, it is often the only vegetable that can be secured at a reasonable cost at certain seasons of the year.

Onions, especially the milder and larger ones, are an excellent and wholesome vegetable, containing small amounts of starch, although their pungent flavor, due to an aromatic oil, makes them so irritating to some stomachs as to be quite indigestible.

Sweet corn, whether fresh or dried, is wholesome, and has a fair degree of nutritive value, as it contains fair amounts of both starch and sugar. It should, however, be very thoroughly chewed and eaten moderately, on account of the thick, firm indigestible husk which surrounds the kernel.

Tomatoes are an exceedingly valuable, though rather recent addition to our dietary. Their fresh, pungent acid is, like the fruit acids, wholesome and beneficial; and they can be preserved or canned without losing any of their flavor. They were at one time denounced as being indigestible, and even as the cause of cancer; but these charges were due to ignorance and distrust of anything new.

Lighter Vegetables, or Paper Foods. The lighter vegetables such as lettuce, celery, spinach, cucumbers, and parsley have, in a previous chapter, been classed with the paper foods. They are all agreeable additions to the diet on account of their fresh taste and pleasant flavor, though they contain little or no nutritive matter.

The Advantages of a Vegetable Garden. Notwithstanding their slight fuel value, there are few more valuable and wholesome elements in the diet than an abundant supply of fresh green vegetables. Everyone who is so situated that he can possibly arrange for it, should have a garden, if only the tiniest patch, and grow them for his own use, both on account of their greater wholesomeness and freshness when so grown, and because of the valuable exercise in the open air, and the enjoyment and interest afforded by their care.

FOOTNOTES:

[10] As vegetables and fruit are bulky and likely to spoil, on the long voyages of sailing vessels before steamships were invented bottles of the juice of limes (a small kind of lemon) were added, instead, to the hard-tack and "salt-horse" of the ship's stores. Because of this custom, the long-voyage merchantmen who carried cargoes round the Horn or the Cape were for years nicknamed "Lime-juicers."

CHAPTER VIII

COOKING

Why We Cook our Food. While some of all classes of food may be eaten raw, yet we have gradually come to submit most of our foods to the heat of a fire, in various ways; this process is known as cooking. While cooking usually wastes a little, and sometimes a good deal, of the fuel value of the food and, if carelessly or stupidly done, may make it less digestible, in the main it makes it both more digestible and safer, though much more expensive. This it does in three ways: by making it taste better; by softening it so as to make it more easily masticated; and by sterilizing it, or destroying any germs or animal parasites which may be in it.

Cooking Improves the Taste of Food. It may seem almost absurd to regard changing the taste of a food as of sufficient importance to justify the expense and trouble of a long process like cooking. Yet this was probably one of the main reasons why cooking came into use in the first place; and it is still one of the most important reasons for continuing it. No one would feel attracted by a plate of slabs of raw meat, with a handful of flour, a raw potato or two, and some green apples; but cook these and you immediately have an appetizing and attractive meal. Any food, to be a thoroughly good food, must "taste good"; otherwise, part of it will fail to be digested, and will sooner or later upset the stomach and clog the appetite.

Cooking Makes Food Easier to Chew and Digest. The second important use of cooking is that it makes food both easier to masticate and easier to digest. As we have seen, it bursts the little coverings of the starchy grains, and makes the tough fibres of grains and roots crisp and brittle, as is well illustrated in the soft, mealy texture of a baked potato, and in the crispness of parched wheat or corn. It coagulates, or curdles, the jelly-like pulp of meat, and the gummy white of the egg, and the sticky gluten of wheat flour, so that they can be ground into tiny pieces between the teeth.

We could hardly eat the different kinds of grains and meals and flours in proper amounts at all, unless they were cooked; indeed they require much longer and more thorough baking, or boiling, than meats. The amount of cooking required should always be borne in mind when counting the cost of a diet, as the fuel, time, and labor consumed in cooking vegetable articles of diet often bring up their expense much more nearly to that of meats than the cost of the raw material in the shops would lead us to expect.

Cooking Sterilizes Food. A third, and probably on the whole, the most valuable and important service rendered by cooking is, that it sterilizes our food and kills any germs, or animal parasites, which may have been in the body of the animal, or in the leaves of the plant, from which it came; or, as is far the commoner and greater danger, may have got on it from dirty or careless handling, or exposure to dust. While it was undoubtedly the great improvement that cooking makes in the taste of food that first led our ancestors--and probably chiefly induces us--to use the process, it is hardly probable that they would have continued to bear the expense, trouble, and numerous discomforts of cooking, had they not noticed this significant fact: that those families and tribes that had the habit of thoroughly cooking their food, suffered least from diseases of the stomach and intestines, and hence lived longer and survived in greater numbers than the "raw fooders." We are perfectly right in spending a good deal of time, care, and thought on cooking, preparing, and serving our food, for we thus lengthen our lives and diminish our sicknesses. Civilized man is far healthier than any known "noble savage," in spite of what poets and story-tellers say to the contrary.

The Three Methods of Cooking. The three[11] chief methods of cooking-- baking, or roasting; boiling, or stewing; and frying--have each their advantages as well as disadvantages. No one of them would be suitable for all kinds of food; and no one of them is to be condemned as unwholesome in itself, if intelligently done; although all of them, if carelessly, or stupidly, carried out, will waste food, and render it less digestible instead of more so. In the main, the methods that are in common use for each particular kind of food, or under each special condition, are reasonable and sensible--the result of hundreds of years of experimenting. The only exceptions are that, on account of its ease and quickness, frying is resorted to rather more frequently than is best; while boiling is more popular than it should be, on account of the small amount of thought and care involved in the process.

Roasting, or Baking. Roasting, or baking, is probably the highest form of the art of cooking, developing the finest flavors, causing less waste of food value, and requiring the greatest skill and care. On general principles, we may say that almost anything which can be roasted or baked, should be roasted or baked.

On the other hand, roasting or baking has the disadvantage of taking a great deal of fuel and of time, and of being exceedingly fatiguing and annoying for the cook, making the labor cost high; and it cannot be used where a meal is needed in a hurry. If the process is carelessly done and carried too far, it may also waste a great deal of the food material, either by burning or scorching, or by the commoner and almost equally wasteful process of turning the whole outside of the roast--particularly in the case of meat--into a hard, tough, leathery substance, which it is almost impossible either to chew or to digest.

Boiling. The advantages of boiling are that it is the easiest of all forms of cookery, and within the grasp of the lowest intelligence; that, on account of keeping the food continually surrounded by water, it leads to less waste and is far less likely than either baking or frying to result in destroying part of the food if not carefully watched; and that it can be used in cooking many cheap, coarse foods, such as the mushes, graham meal, corn meal, hominy, potatoes, cabbages, turnips, etc., which furnish the bulk of our food.

On the other hand, from the point of view of fuel used, it is the most expensive of all forms of cooking; and unless a fire is being kept up for other purposes, which allows boiling or stewing to go on on the back of the stove as an "extra," without additional expense, careful experiments have shown that the prolonged boiling needed by many of these cheaper and coarser foods, especially such as are recommended by most diet reformers, brings their total cost up to that of bread, milk, eggs, sugar, and the cheaper cuts of meat,--all of which are more wholesome and more appetizing foods.

The supposed saving in boiling meat, that you get two courses, soup and meat, out of one joint, is imaginary; for, as we have seen, the soup or water in which meat has been boiled contains little, or nothing, of the fuel value, or nourishing part of the meat; and all the flavor that is saved in this is lost by the boiled meat, rendering it not only much less appetizing, but also less digestible. You cannot have the flavor of your food in two places at once. If you save it in the soup, you lose it from the meat.

Frying. The chief advantages of frying are its marked saving of time, of fuel, and of discomfort to the cook; it also develops the appetizing flavors of the food to a very high degree. A wholesome, appetizing meal can be prepared by frying, much more quickly than by either baking or boiling, and with less than half the fuel expense.

The drawbacks of frying come chiefly from unintelligent and careless methods of applying it. It is somewhat wasteful of food material, particularly of meats; although, if the fat which is fried out in the process can be used in other cooking, or turned into a gravy, a good deal of this waste can be avoided. As, in frying, some form of fat has to be used to keep the food from burning, this fat is apt to form a coating over the surface and, if used in excessive amounts, at too low a temperature, may soak deeply into the food, thus coating over every particle of it with a thick, water-proof film, which prevents the juices of the stomach and the upper part of the bowel from attacking and digesting it. This undesirable result, however, can be entirely avoided by having both the pan and the melted fat which it contains, very hot, before the steak, chop, potatoes, or buckwheat cakes are put into the pan. When this is done, the heat of the pan and of the boiling fat instantly sears over the whole surface of the piece of food, and forms a coating which prevents the further penetration of the fat. Quick frying is, as a rule, a safe and wholesome form of cooking. Slow frying, which means stewing in melted grease for twenty or thirty minutes, is one of the most effective ways ever invented of spoiling good food and ruining digestion.

Why Every One should Learn how to Cook. Every boy and every girl ought to know how to cook. Cooking is a most interesting art, and a knowledge of it is a valuable part of a good education. Everybody would find such a knowledge exceedingly useful at some time in his life; and most of us, all our lives long. As a life-saving accomplishment, it is much more valuable than knowing how to swim. Every schoolhouse of more than five rooms should have a kitchen and a lunch room as part of its equipment, and classes should take turns in cooking and serving lunches for the rest of the children.[12]

FOOTNOTES:

[11] For meats a fourth method may be used--broiling, which for flavor and wholesomeness is superior to any other, but requires a special and rather expensive type of clear, hot fire and a high degree of skill.

[12] Whenever lunches are brought by children, or the school-lunch is a problem, if possible equip a spare room with a gas or a coal stove, sink, tables, chairs, necessary dishes, etc., and let classes under direction of teacher take turns in purchasing food supplies for lunch; cooking and serving lunch; planning dietaries with reference to balanced nutrition, digestibility, and

cheapness; washing pots, pans, and dishes; cleaning kitchen; protecting and storing foods; finding risks of spoiling, contamination, infection, fly-visiting; and practicing other forms of kitchen hygiene.

CHAPTER IX

OUR DRINK

FILLING THE BOILER OF THE BODY-ENGINE

The Need of Water in the Body-Engine. If you have ever taken a long railway journey, you will remember that, about every two or three hours, you would stop longer than usual at some station, or switch, for the engine to take in water. No matter how briskly the fire burns in the furnace, or how much good coal you may shovel into it, if there be no water in the boiler above it to expand and make steam, the engine will do no work. And an abundant supply of water is just as necessary in our own bodies, although not used in just the same way as in the engine.

The singular thing about water, both in a locomotive and in our own bodies is that, absolutely necessary as it is, it is neither burned up nor broken down in any way, in making the machine go; so that it gives off no energy, as our food does, but simply changes its form slightly. Exactly the same amount of water, to the ounce, or even the teaspoonful, that is poured into the boiler of an engine, is given off through its funnel and escape-pipes in the form of steam; and precisely the same amount of water which we pour into our stomachs will reappear on the surface of the body again in the form of the vapor from the lungs, the perspiration from the skin, and the water from the kidneys. It goes completely through the engine, or the body, enables the one to work and the other to live, and yet comes out unchanged.

Just how water works in the engine we know--the heat from the furnace changes it into steam, which means that heat expands it, or makes it fill more space. This swelling pushes forward the cylinder that starts the wheels of the engine. The next puff gives them another whirl, and in a few minutes the big locomotive is puffing steadily down the track.

Water is Necessary to Life. Just how water works in the body we do not know, as most of it is not even turned into steam or vapor. But this much we do know, that life cannot exist in the absence of water. Odd as it may seem to us at first sight, ninety-five, yes, ninety-nine per cent of our body cells are water-animals, and can live and grow only when literally swimming in water.

The scaly cells on the surface of our skin, our hair, and the tips of our nails are the only parts of us that live in air. In fact, over five-sixths of the weight and bulk of our bodies is made up of water. Some one has quaintly, but truthfully, described the human body as composed of a few pounds of charcoal, a bushel of air, half a peck of lime, and a couple of handfuls of salt dissolved in four buckets of water. The reason why nearly all our foods, as we have seen, contain such large amounts of water is that they, also, are the results of life--the tissues and products of plants or animals.

Water Frees the Body from Waste Substances. Water in the body, then, is necessary to life itself. But another most important use is to wash out all the waste substances from the different organs and tissues and carry them to the liver, the kidneys, the lungs, and the skin, where they can be burned up and got rid of. We must keep our bodies well flushed with water, just as we should keep a free current of water flowing through our drain-pipes and sewers.

It Keeps the Body from Getting Over-heated. In summer time, or in hot climates the year round, an abundant supply of water is of great importance in keeping the body from becoming overheated, by pouring itself out on the skin in the form of perspiration, and cooling us by evaporation, as we shall see in the chapter on the skin.

The Meaning of Thirst. None of us who has ever been a mile or more away from a well, or brook, on a hot summer's day needs to be told how necessary water is, for comfort as well as for health. The appetite which we have developed for it--thirst, as we call it--is the most tremendous and powerful craving that we can feel, and the results of water starvation are as serious and as quick in coming as is the keenness of our thirst. Men in fairly good condition, if they are at rest, and not exposed to hardship, and have plenty of water to drink, can survive without food for from two to four weeks; but if deprived of water, they will perish in agony in from two to three days.

We should Drink Three Pints of Water a Day. Although all our foods, either as we find them in the state of nature, or as they come on the table cooked and prepared for eating, contain large quantities of water, this is not enough for the needs of the body; to keep in good health we must also drink in some form about three pints, or six glassfuls, of water in the course of the day. Part of this goes, as you will remember (p. 16), to dissolve the food so that it can be readily absorbed by our body cells in the process of digestion.

WHERE OUR DRINKING WATER COMES FROM

Water Contained in our Food is Pure. Seeing that five-sixths of our food is water, it is clearly of the greatest importance that that water should be pure. That part of our water supply which we get in and with our foods is fortunately, for the most part, almost perfectly pure, having been specially filtered by the plants or animals which originally drank it, or having been boiled in the process of cooking.

Water is Always in Motion. The part of our water supply which we take directly, in the form of drinking water, is, however, unfortunately anything but free from danger of impurities. The greatest difficulty with water is that it will not "stay put"--it is continually on the move. The same perpetual circulation, with change of form, but without loss of substance, which is taking place in the engine and in our bodies, is taking place in the world around us. The water from the ocean, the lakes, and the rivers is continually evaporating under the heat of the sun and rising in the form of vapor, or invisible steam, into the air. There it becomes cooler, and forms the clouds; and when these are cooled a little more, the vapor changes into drops of water and pours down as rain, or, if the droplets freeze, as snow or hail. The rain falls upon the leaves of the trees and the spears of the grass, or the thirsty plowed ground, soaks down into the soil and "seeps" or drains gradually into the streams and rivers, and down these into the lakes and oceans, to be again pumped up by the sun. All we can do is to catch what we need of it, "on the run," somewhere in the earthy part of its circuit.

Why our Drinking Water is Likely to be Impure. Every drop of water that we drink or use, fell somewhere on the surface of the earth, in the form of rain or snow; and if we wish to find out whether it is pure and safe, we must trace its course through the soil, or the streams, from the point where it fell. Our drinking water has literally washed "all outdoors" before it reaches us, and what it may have picked up in that washing makes the possibilities of its danger.

As it falls from the skies, it is perfectly pure--except in large cities or manufacturing centres, where rain water contains small amounts of soot, smoke-acids, and dust, but even these are in such small amounts as to be practically harmless. But the moment it reaches the ground, it begins to soak up something out of everything that it touches; and here our dangers begin.

Risks from Leaf Mould. Practically the whole surface of the earth is covered with some form of vegetation--grass, trees, or other green plants. These dying down and decaying year after year, form a layer of vegetable mould such as you can readily scratch up on the surface of the ground in a forest or old meadow; this is known as leaf mould, or humus. As the water soaks through this mould, it becomes loaded with decaying vegetable matter, which it carries with it down into the soil. Most of this, fortunately, is comparatively harmless to the human digestion. But some of this vegetable matter, such as we find in the water from bogs or swamps, or even heavy forests, will sometimes upset the digestion; hence, the natural dislike that we have for water with a marshy, or "weedy," taste.

Nature's Filter-Bed. When, however, this peaty water soaks on down through the grass, roots, and leaf mold, into the soil, it comes in contact with Nature's great filter-bed--the second place in the circuit where the water is again made perfectly pure. This filter-bed consists of a layer of more or less spongy, porous soil, or earth, swarming with millions of tiny vegetable germs known as bacteria. These eagerly pick out all the decaying vegetable substances of the water and feed upon them, changing them into harmless carbon dioxid water, and small amounts of ammonia. Not only will this filter-bed, or spongy mat of bacteria, burn up and remove all traces of vegetable decay, but if the rain happens to have soaked through the decaying body of a bird or animal or insect, the bacteria will just as eagerly feed upon these animal substances and change them into harmless gases and salts.[13]

By the time the rain water has reached the deeper layers of the soil, it is again perfectly pure and has also, in seeping through the soil, picked up certain mineral salts (such as calcium, sodium, and magnesium) which are of use in the body; so that in an open or thinly settled country, the water in streams, rivers, and lakes is usually fairly pure and quite wholesome. That is why, in ancient times, the great majority of villages and towns and camps were situated on the bank of some stream, where a supply of water could easily be obtained.

CAUSES AND DANGERS OF POLLUTED WATER

Wells--the Oldest Method of Supplying Water. It was long ago discovered that, by digging pits or holes in the ground, the rain water, in its steady flow toward the streams and lakes, could be caught or trapped, and that if the pit were made deep enough, a sufficient amount would accumulate during the winter or spring to last well on into the summer, unless the season were unusually dry. These pits, or water traps, are our familiar wells, from which most of our water supply, except in the large cities, is still taken. These wells were naturally dug, or sunk, as near as might be to the house, so as to shorten the distance that the water had to be carried; and from this arose their chief and greatest source of danger.

The Danger to Wells from Household Waste. Every house has, like our bodies, a certain amount of waste, which must be got rid of. Some of this material can, of course, be fed to pigs and chickens, and in that way disposed of. But the simplest and easiest thing to do with the watery parts of the household waste is to take them to the back door and throw them out on the ground, while table-scraps and other garbage are thrown into the long grass, or bushes--a method which is still, unfortunately, pursued in a great many houses in the country and the suburbs of towns. If the area over which they are thrown is large enough, and particularly if the soil is porous and well covered with vegetation, nature's filter-bed--the soil, the bacteria, and the roots of the grass and other plants combined--will purify a surprising amount of waste; but there is always the danger, particularly in the wet weather of spring and of late fall, that the soil will become charged with more of these waste matters than the bacteria can destroy, and that these waste poisons will be washed down in the rain water right into the pit, or trap, which has been dug for it--the well.

The Danger from Outbuildings. This danger is further increased by the fact that for the same reason--the vital need of plenty of water for all living creatures--the hen coop, the pig pen, the cow stable, and the horse barn are all likely to be built clustering around this same well. If the fertilizer from these places is, as it should be in all intelligent farming, protected from the rain so as not to have all its strength washed out of it, and removed and spread on the soil at frequent intervals, the well may even yet escape contamination; but the chances are very strongly against it. If you will figure out that a well drains the surface soil in every direction for a distance from ten to thirty times its own depth, and that the average well is about twenty-five feet deep, you can readily see what a risk of contaminating the well is caused by every barn, outhouse, or pen within from sixty to a hundred and fifty yards from its mouth.

Every well from which drinking water is taken should be at least fifty, and better, a hundred and fifty, yards away from any stable, outhouse, or barn; or set well up-hill from it, so that all drainage runs away from its basin. This, of course, is possible only in the country, or in villages or small towns, where houses have plenty of ground about them. Consequently, the health laws of most cities and states forbid the use of shallow wells for drinking purposes in cities of over 10,000 population.

Causes which Produce Pure Well Water. Occasionally a well will be driven through a layer of rock or hard water-proof clay, before the water-bearing layer of soil, or sand, is struck, so that its water will be drawn, not from the rain that falls on the surface of the ground immediately about it, but from that which has fallen somewhere at a considerable distance and filtered down through the soil. This water, on account of the many, many layers of soil through which it has filtered, and the long distance it has come, is usually fairly pure, so far as animal or vegetable impurities are concerned, though it is apt to have become too strong in certain salty and mineral substances, which give it a taste of salt, or iron, or sulphur. If, however, it is free from these salty substances, it makes a very pure and wholesome drinking water; and if the upper part of the well shaft be lined with bricks and cement, so that the surface water cannot leak into it, it may be used with safety for drinking purposes even in the heart of a city.

The Greatest Single Danger to Well Water. The greatest single danger to the purity of well water is the privy vault. This is doubly dangerous, first, because it is dug below the level at which the bacteria in the soil are most abundant and active, so that they cannot attack and break up its contents; and the impurities, therefore, are gradually washed down by the rain water into the soil, unchanged, and seep directly into the well. The other reason is that its contents may contain the germs of serious diseases, particularly typhoid fever and other bowel troubles. These germs and their poisons would usually be destroyed by the bacteria of the soil, if not poured out in too large quantities; but in the privy vault they escape their attack, and so are carried on with the slow leakage of water into the well; then those who use that water are very liable to have typhoid fever and other serious diseases.

Early Methods of Prevention. On account of these filth-dangers, it began, a century or so ago, to be the custom in cleanly and thoughtful households to provide, first, ditches, and then, lines of pipes, made out of hollow wood or baked clay, and later of iron, called drains, through which all the watery parts of household wastes could be carried away and poured out at some distance from the house. Then toilets, or flush-closets, were built, and this kind of waste was carried completely away from the house, and beyond danger of contaminating the wells.

How Streams were Contaminated. For a time this seemed to end the danger, as the waste was soaked up by the soil, and eaten by its hungry bacteria and drunk up again by the roots of plants. But when ten or a dozen houses began to combine and run their drain-pipes together into a large drain called a sewer, then this could not open upon the surface of the ground, but had to be run into some stream, or brook, in order to be carried away. As cities and towns, which had been obliged to give up their wells, were beginning to collect the water from these same brooks and streams in reservoirs and deliver it in pipes to all their houses, it can be easily seen that we had simply exchanged one danger for another.

The Loss of Life from Typhoid Fever. For a time, indeed, it looked as if the new danger were the greater of the two, because, when the typhoid germs were washed into a well, they poisoned or infected only one, or at most two or three, families who used the water from that well. But when they were carried into a stream which was dammed to form a reservoir to supply a town with water, then the whole population of the town might become infected. A great many epidemics of typhoid fever occurred in just this way, before people realized how great this danger was. Simply from the pouring of the wastes from one or two typhoid fever cases into the streams leading into the water reservoir used by a town, five hundred, a thousand, or even three or four thousand cases of typhoid have developed within a few weeks, with from one hundred to five hundred deaths.

In 1891-92 typhoid fever broke out in Schenectady on the Mohawk River. Following this, Cohoes and West Troy, which drew their water supply from the Mohawk below Schenectady, and Albany, which drew its supply from the Hudson below the mouth of the Mohawk, suffered from typhoid epidemics; while Waterford and Troy, which drew their supplies from the Hudson above the mouth of the Mohawk, and the river towns that, like Lansingburgh, drew from other sources, entirely escaped the infection.

In fact, even to-day, when these dangers are better understood, and while most of our big cities are getting fairly clear of typhoid, so ignorant and careless are the smaller towns, villages, and private houses all over the United States, that over 35,000 deaths[14] from typhoid fever occur every year in a country which prides itself upon its cleanliness and its intelligence. This means, too, that there are at least half a million people sick of the disease, and in bed or utterly prevented from working, for from five to fifteen weeks each. All of which frightful loss of human life and human labor, to say nothing of the grief, bereavement, and anxiety of the two million or more families and relatives of these typhoid victims, is due to eating dirt and drinking filth. Dirt is surely the most expensive thing there is, instead of the cheapest.

METHODS OF OBTAINING PURE WATER

Wise Planning and Spending of Money is Necessary. If our city wells are defiled by manure heaps and vault-privies, and our streams by sewage, where are we to turn for pure water? All that is required is foresight and a little intelligent planning and wise spending of money. Of course the community must take hold of the problem, through a Board of Health, or Health Officer, appointed for the purpose; and this is why questions of health are coming to play such an important part in legislation, and even in politics. No matter how fast a city is growing or how much money its inhabitants are making, if it has an impure water supply or a bad sewage system, there will be disease and death, suffering and unhappiness among its people, which no amount of money can make up for. Cleanliness is not only next to godliness, but one of the most useful forms of it; and a city can afford to spend money liberally to secure it--in fact, it is the best investment a city can make.

Artesian and Deep Wells. The earliest, and still the most eagerly sought-for, source of pure water supply is springs or deep wells, such as we have referred to. Both of these are fed by rain water which has fallen somewhere upon the surface of the earth. As the layers of earth or rock, of which the crust of the earth is made up, do not run level, or horizontal, but are tilted and tipped in all directions, this rain water soaks down until it reaches one of these sloping layers that is so hard, or tough, as to be waterproof, and then runs along over its surface in a sort of underground stream. If anywhere in the course of this stream a very deep well shaft is driven right down through the soil until it strikes the surface of this sloping layer of rock, then the water will rise in this shaft to the level of the highest point from which it is running.

If this highest point of the waterproof layer be many miles away, up in the hills above the surface of the ground where the well is dug, then the water will rise to the surface and sometimes even spout twenty, thirty, or fifty feet above it. This forms what is known as a gushing, or artesian, well (from Artois, a province in France, in which such wells were first commonly used) and furnishes a very pure and valuable source of water supply. If it rises only twenty, thirty, or fifty feet in the well-shaft, but keeps flowing in at a sufficient rate, then we get what is known as a "living," or permanent well, and this also is a very valuable and pure source of water supply.

Springs. Springs are formed on the same plan as the deep well, but with the difference that the waterproof layer on top of which the water is running either crops out on the surface again, lower down the mountain, or folds upon itself and comes up again to the surface some distance away from the mountain chain, out on the level. This is why springs are usually found in or near mountainous or hilly regions. If the water of a spring has gone deep enough into, or far enough through, the layers of the earth, it may, like water of some of the artesian wells, contain certain salts and minerals, particularly soda, sulphur, and iron. Such springs are often highly valued as mineral water, healing springs, or baths, partly because of these salts, partly on account of their peculiar taste. Most of the virtues ascribed to mineral waters or springs are due, however, to their pure water, and its cleansing effects internally and externally when freely used.

Springs are among the most highly prized sources of water supply, because they have gone underground sufficiently deep to become well filtered and cooled to a low temperature, and usually not far enough to become too heavily loaded with salts or minerals like the waters of the deep wells. It must, however, be remembered that they also come from rain-water, and that in hilly or broken regions the source of that rain water may be the surface of the ground only a few hundred yards up the hill or mountain, and impurities there may affect it. Much of the delightful sparkle of spring water is due, as in the case of the popular soda water, to the presence of carbon dioxid, only in spring water it is produced by the decomposition of vegetable matter in it. As springs usually break out in a hollow or at the foot of a hill, unless carefully closed in they are quite liable to contamination from rain water from the surrounding surface of the ground. Where springs of a sufficient size can be reached, or a sufficiently "live" series of deep wells can be bored, these furnish a safe source of water supply for cities. But of course not more than one city in five or ten is so favored.

Mountain Reservoirs. Two other methods of securing a water supply are now generally adopted. One is to pick out some stream up in the hills or mountains, within fifteen miles or so of the city, and put in a dam, thus making a reservoir, or to enlarge some lake which already exists there. At the same time, the entire valley, or slope of the mountain, which this stream or lake drains of its surface water, is bought up by the Government, or turned into a forest reserve, so that no houses can be built or settlement of any kind permitted upon it. It can still be used for lumber supply, for pastures, and, within reasonable limits, for a great public hunting and fishing reserve and camping resort.

Almost every intelligent and farsighted town, which has not springs or deep wells, is looking toward the acquirement of some such area as this for its source of pure water. Many great cities go from thirty to fifty miles, and some even a hundred and fifty miles, in order to reach such a source, carrying the water into the city in a huge water-pipe, or aqueduct. These cities find that the millions of dollars saved by the prevention of death and disease amount to many times the cost of such a system, while the water rents gladly paid by both private houses and manufacturing establishments give good interest on the investment. Any town can afford to go a mile for every thousand of its population for such a source of water supply as this; and secure, gratis, a valuable forest preserve, public park, and beauty spot.[15]

Filtration. The other method, which has to be adopted by cities situated on level plains, or at the mouths of great rivers, is to take the water of some lake, or river, as far out in the former, or as high up the latter, as possible, and purify it by filtration. This can be done at a moderate expense by preparing great settling-basins and filter-beds. The first are great pools or small lakes, into which the water is run and held until most of the mud and coarser dirt has settled or sunk. Then this clear water above the sediment is run on to great beds, first of gravel, then of coarse sand, then of fine sand; and if these beds are large enough, and frequently changed and cleaned, so that they do not become clogged, and the process is carried out slowly, the water, when it comes through the last bed, is pure enough to drink safely.[16]

One of these sources of a safe and wholesome water-supply--the deep flowing well, or spring; the water shut up in the mountains in its lake or reservoir; or the slow filter-bed--should be used by every intelligent and progressive town of more than a thousand inhabitants.

Sewage and its Disposal. At the same time, while seeking a source of water-supply far removed from any possibility of contagion, we must not neglect the other end of the problem, the protecting of our rivers and lakes from pollution so far as possible; for the water from these must necessarily be used by thousands of people along their banks, either directly, or in the form of shallow wells, sunk not far from the water's edge. Moreover, so foul are many of our rivers and streams becoming in thickly settled regions that fish can no longer live in them, and it is hardly safe to bathe in them.[17] Fortunately, however, a great deal of the worst contamination can be prevented by using modern methods of disposing of sewage, such as filter-beds and sewage farms. All of these methods use the bacteria of the soil, or crops growing in it, to eat up the waste and thus purify the sewage.

HOME METHODS OF PURIFYING WATER

Boiling. Where the water that you are obliged to drink is not known to be pure, then it can be made quite safe for drinking purposes by the simple process of boiling it for about ten or fifteen minutes. But this, except in travelling or in emergencies, is a lazy, slipshod substitute for pure water, and extremely unsatisfactory as well; for the boiling drives off all its air and other gases, and throws down most of the salts, so that boiled water has a flat, insipid taste. These salts, although sometimes regarded as impurities, are not such in any true sense; for the lime and soda especially are of considerable value in the body, so that boiled or sterilized water is neither a pleasant nor a wholesome permanent drink. Instead of boiling the water, get to work to protect your own well from filth of all sorts, if you drink well water; or, if not, to help the Board of Health to agitate, and keep on agitating, until something is done to compel your selectmen or City Council to secure a pure supply.

Domestic Filters. Much the same must be said of private or domestic filters. These are, at best, temporary substitutes, and should not be depended upon for permanent use. Many of them are made to sell rather than to purify, and will remove only the larger or mechanical impurities from the water. Others, while they work well at first, are exceedingly likely to become clogged, when the tendency is to punch at them to make them work faster, thus either poking a hole through them or cracking the filter-shell, so that a stream of water flows steadily through, just as impure as when it entered. Private filters, like boiling water, are only temporary ways of meeting conditions which ought not to be allowed to exist at all in civilized communities, or in your own homes.

A score of court decisions in all parts of the world have now held that the water company is legally responsible for all avoidable pollution of public water-supplies, and nine tenths of pollutions are avoidable.

FOOTNOTES:

[13] These gases and salts are eagerly sucked up by the roots of plants, so that the soil bacteria are our best friends, changing poisonous decaying things into harmless plant-foods. They are the chief secret of the fertility of a soil; and the more there are of them the richer a soil is.

[14] This makes fourteen times as many deaths from typhoid in proportion to the population as occur in Germany.

[15] New York City, for instance, goes forty miles up into the hills to the great Croton reservoir for its water supply; and as this is proving insufficient, is preparing to go ninety-five miles up into the Ramapo Hills to secure control of a whole country-side for a permanent source of supply. Portland, Oregon, nearly twenty years ago, with then a population of some 75,000, built an aqueduct sixty miles up into the mountains to a lake on the side of Mt. Hood, and has reaped the advantages of its foresight ever since, in a low death rate and a rapid growth (200,000 in 1910), as well as a financial profit on its investment. Los Angeles, California, is preparing to build an aqueduct a hundred and thirty miles, and tunnel two mountain ranges in order to reach an inexhaustible supply of water.

[16] Of late, currents of electricity are passed through the water (setting free oxygen or ozone) which make the purifying of it much more rapid and complete.

It is, however, often considered safer to pass the water through still another filter bed, consisting of layers of charcoal, which has the power of gathering oxygen in its pores, to attack and oxidize, or burn up, the remaining impurities in the water. A sort of scum forms over the surface of the last and finest bed of sand or charcoal, and if this scum is not too frequently removed, though it makes the filtering slower, the water comes out purer. On examining this scum, we find it to consist of a thick mat of our old friends, the purifying bacteria of the soil. So that the last step of our artificial filtration is simply an imitation of nature's great filter-bed.

[17] Several streams emptying into the Ohio River from a thickly settled region are said to be actually pumped out into waterworks systems, used for drinking, washing, and manufacturing, and run back into the river again through sewers by the different cities along its banks, at such frequent intervals that every drop of water in them passes through waterworks systems and sewers three times before it reaches the mouth of the stream.

CHAPTER X

BEVERAGES, ALCOHOL, AND TOBACCO

The Popularity of Beverages. For some curious reason, the habit has grown up of taking a large part of the six glasses of water that we require daily in the form of mixtures known as beverages. These beverages are always much more expensive than pure water; are often quite troublesome to secure and prepare; have little, or no, food value; are of doubtful value even in small amounts; and injurious in large ones. Why they should ever have come into such universal use, in all races and in all ages of the world, is one of the standing puzzles of human nature. They practically all consist of from ninety to ninety-eight per cent of water, the food elements that may be added to them being in such trifling amounts as to be practically of no value. They serve no known useful purpose in the body, save as a means of introducing the water which they contain; and yet mankind has used them ever since the dawn of history.

We Have no Natural Appetite for Beverages. It is a most striking fact that, although these beverages have been drunk by the race for centuries, we have never developed an instinct or natural appetite for them! No child ever yet was born with an appetite or natural liking for beer or whiskey; and very few children really like the taste of tea or coffee the first time, although they soon learn to drink them on account of the sugar and cream in them. Thus, nature has clearly marked them off from all the real foods on our tables, showing that they are not essential to either life or health; and that they are absolutely unnecessary, and almost always harmful in childhood and during the period of growth. If no child ever drank alcohol until he really craved it, as he craves milk, sugar, and bread and butter, there would be no drunkards in the world. Our other food-instincts have shown themselves worthy to be trusted--why not trust this one, and let these beverages, especially alcohol, absolutely alone?

Statistics from the alcoholic wards of our great hospitals show that of those who become drunkards, nearly ninety per cent begin to drink before they are twenty years old. Of that ninety per cent, over two-thirds took their first drink, not because they felt any craving for it, or even thought it would taste good, but because they saw others doing it; or thought it would be a "manly" thing to do; or were afraid that they would be laughed at if they didn't! Whatever vices and bad habits our natural appetites, and so-called "animal instincts," may lead us into, drunkenness is not one of them.

This striking hint on the part of nature, that alcoholic beverages are unnecessary, is fully confirmed by the overwhelming majority of hundreds of tests which have been made in the laboratory, showing clearly that, while these beverages may give off trifling amounts of energy in the body, their real effects and the sole reason for their use are their stimulating, or their discomfort-deadening (narcotic) effect. And the more carefully we study them, the heavier we find the price that has to be paid for any temporary relief or enjoyment which they may seem to give.

Tea, Coffee, and Cocoa. The "weakest" and most commonly used of these beverages or amusement foods, are tea, coffee, and cocoa. These have an agreeable taste, mildly stimulate the nervous system, and, when used in moderation by adults, seldom do much harm. To a small percentage of individuals, who are specially sensitive to their effects, they seem to act as mild poison-foods, much in the same way as strawberries, cheese, or lobsters do to others.

Tea is made from the green leaves of a shrub growing in hilly districts in China, Japan, and Southern India. The finer and more delicately flavored brands are from the young leaves, shoots, and flowers of the plant; while the coarser and cheaper are from the old leaves, stalks, and even twigs--the latter containing the most tannin, which, as we shall see, is the most injurious element in tea.

Coffee is made from the seeds of a cherry-like berry growing upon a shrub, or low tree, on tropical hillsides. The bulk of our supply comes from South America, and is known as "Rio" coffee, from Rio Janeiro, the port in Brazil from which most of it is shipped. That from the East Indies is known as Java, and that from Arabia as Mocha; though these last two are now but little more than trade-names for certain finer varieties of coffee, no matter where grown.

Cocoa and chocolate are made from the bean-like seeds of a small tree growing in the tropics and, in cake, or solid, form, contain considerable amounts of fat, and usually sugar and vanilla, which have been added to them to improve their flavor. As, however, only a teaspoonful or so of the powdered cocoa, or chocolate, goes to make a cupful, the actual food value of cocoa or chocolate, unless made with milk, is not much greater than that of tea or coffee with cream and sugar. They contain less caffein than either tea or coffee, but are liable to clog rather than to increase the appetite for other foods.

Effects of Tea, Coffee, and Cocoa. Though the flavors of tea, coffee, and cocoa are so different, they all depend for their effect upon a spicy-tasting substance, called caffein from its having been first separated out of coffee. The caffein of tea is sometimes called thein, and that of cocoa theobromin; but they are all practically the same substance. Part of the taste of these beverages is due to the caffein, but the special flavor of each is given by spicy oils and other substances which it contains. Caffein acts as a mild stimulant both to the nervous system and brain, and to the heart; as is shown by the way in which tea or coffee will wake us up or refresh us when tired, or, if drunk too late at night, keep us from going to sleep. If used in large amounts, especially if taken as a substitute for food, tea and coffee upset the nervous system and disturb the heart, and produce an unwholesome craving for more.

Their chief value lies in the hot water they contain, which has been sterilized by boiling, while its heat assists the process of digestion; and in the fact that their agreeable taste sometimes gives us an appetite and enables us to eat more of less highly flavored foods, like bread, crackers, potatoes, or rice, than we would without them. They are, also, usually taken with cream, or milk, or sugar, which are real foods and bring their fuel value up to about half that of skimmed milk. So far as they stimulate the appetite and increase the amount of food eaten, they are beneficial; but when taken as a substitute for real food, they are most injurious. A cup of coffee, for instance, makes a very poor breakfast to start the day on; for although it gives you a comforting sense of having eaten something warm and satisfying, it contains very little real food, and soon leaves you feeling empty and tired; just as an engine would give out if you put a handful of shavings into its fire-box, and expected it to do four hours' work on them.

The most disturbing effects of tea and coffee upon the digestion are due to the tannin which they contain if boiled too long, especially in the case of tea. This tannin, fortunately, will not dissolve in water except by prolonged boiling or steeping; so that if tea is made by pouring boiling water over the tea leaves and pouring it off again as soon as it has reached the desired strength and flavor, and coffee by being just brought to a boil and then not allowed to stand more than ten or fifteen minutes before use, no injurious amounts of tannin will be found in them. Tea, made by prolonged stewing on the back of the stove, owes its bitter, puckery taste to tannin, and is better suited for tanning leather than for putting into the human stomach.

Boys and girls up to fifteen or sixteen years of age are much better off without tea, coffee, or cocoa; for they need no artificial stimulants to their appetites, while at the same time their nervous systems are more liable to injury from the harmful effects of over-stimulation. If the beverages are taken at all, they should be taken very weak, and with plenty of milk and cream as well as sugar.

ALCOHOL

How Alcohol is Made. The most dangerous addition that man has ever made to the water which he drinks is alcohol. It is made by the action of the yeast plant on wet sugar or starch--a process called fermentation. Usually the sugar or starch is in the form of the juice of fruits; or is a pulp, or mash, made from crushed grains like barley, corn, or rye. As the spores of this yeast plant are floating about almost everywhere in the air, all that is usually necessary is to let some fruit juice or grain pulp stand at moderate warmth, exposed to the air, when it will begin to "sour," or ferment.

Wine. When the yeast plant is set to work in a tub or vat of grape juice, it attacks the fruit sugar contained in the juice, and splits it up into alcohol and carbon dioxid, so that the juice becomes bubbly and frothy from the gas. When from seven to fifteen per cent of alcohol has been produced, the liquid is called wine. It contains, besides alcohol, some unchanged fruit sugar, fruit acids, and some other products of fermentation (known as ethers and aldehydes), which give each kind of wine its special flavor.

Beer, Ale, and Cider. If the yeast germ be set to work in a pulp or mash of crushed barley or wheat, the starch of which has been partly turned into sugar by malting, it breaks up the sugar into alcohol and carbon dioxid. When it has brewed enough of the starch to produce somewhere from four to eight per cent of alcohol, then the liquid, which still contains about three or four per cent of a starch-sugar called maltose, is called beer, or ale. It is usually flavored with hops to give it a bitter taste and make it keep better. If the same process be carried out in apple juice, we get the well known hard cider with its biting taste.

Whiskey, Brandy, and Rum. When left to itself, the process of fermentation in most of these sugary or starchy liquids will come to a standstill after a while, because the alcohol, when it reaches a certain strength in the liquid, is, like all other toxins, or poisons produced by germs, a poison also to the germ that produces it. The yeast-bacteria probably produce alcohol as a poison to kill off other germs which compete with them for their share of the sugar or starch. So even the origin of this curious drug-food shows its harmful character. We should hardly pick out the poison produced by one germ to kill another germ as likely to make a useful and wholesome food.

If man had been content to leave this fermentation process to nature, it is probable that many of the worst effects of alcohol would never have been heard of. But these lighter forms of alcoholic drinks did not satisfy the unnatural cravings which they had themselves created. Some people never can leave even bad-enough alone. So man, with an ingenuity which might have been much better used, sought a way of getting a liquor which would contain more alcohol than nature, unaided, could be made to brew in it. A little experimenting showed that the alcohol in fermenting juices was lighter than water; so that by gently heating the fermenting mass, the alcohol would evaporate and pass off as vapor, with a little of the steam from the water. Then, by catching this vapor in a closed vessel and pouring cold water over the outside of the vessel, it could be condensed again in the form of a clear, brownish fluid of burning taste, containing nearly fifty per cent of alcohol, instead of the original five or six.

This evaporated or distilled mixture of alcohol and water, if made from a mash of corn, wheat, rye, or potatoes, is called whiskey; if from fruit-juice, brandy. A similar liquor, made out of fermented rice, is known as arrack in India, or sak?in Japan; and the liquor made from fermented molasses is called rum.

Alcohol not a True Food, but a Drug. The much disputed question as to whether alcohol is a food or not, is really of little or no practical importance. It is quite true, as might be expected, from its close relation to sugar and the readiness, for instance, with which it will burn in an alcohol lamp or stove, that alcohol, in small amounts, is capable of being burned in the body, thus giving it energy. This may give it a certain limited value in some forms of sickness, as, for instance, in certain fevers and infections, when the stomach does not seem to be able to digest food. But here it acts as a medicine rather than as a true food and, like all other medicines, should be used only under skilled medical advice and control. For practical purposes, any trifling food value it may have is more than offset by its later poisonous and disturbing effects and, secondly, by its enormous expensiveness.

The greatest amount of alcohol that could be consumed in the body at all safely would barely supply one-tenth of the total fuel value needed; and if any one were to attempt to supply the body with energy by the use of alcohol, he would be blind drunk before he had taken one-third of the amount required. From the point of view of expense alone, to take alcohol for food is like killing buffalos for their tongues and letting the rest of the carcass go to waste, as the Indians and pioneer hunters of the plains used to do. It never has more than a fraction of the food value of the grain or fruit out of which it was made; and the amount of nutriment that it contains costs ten times as much as it would in any of the staple foods.

Moreover, when it is taken with an ordinary supply of food, it is found that, for every ounce of alcohol burned in the body, a similar amount of the other food is prevented from being consumed, and probably goes to waste, owing to the harmful effects of alcohol upon digestion. Therefore, to talk of alcohol as a food is really absurd.

The Effect of Alcohol on Digestion. It has been urged by some that alcohol increases the appetite, and enables one to digest larger amounts of food. The early experiments seemed to support this claim by showing that alcohol, well diluted, and in moderate amounts, increased appetite and the flow of the gastric juice. When the experiments were carried a little further, however, it was clearly shown that its presence in the stomach and intestines, in such amounts as would result from a glass of beer, or one or two glasses of claret-wine with a meal, interfered with the later stages of digestion, so that the later harmful effects overbalanced any earlier good effects.

Its Effect on the Temperature of the Body. Another claim urged in its favor was that it warmed the body and protected it against cold. It ought to have been easy for any one with a sense of humor to judge the value of this claim by the fact that it was equally highly commended by its users as a means of keeping them cool in hot weather. Its supposed effects in the case of both heat and cold were due to the same fact: it deadened the nerves for a time to whatever sense of discomfort one might then be suffering from, but made no change whatever in the condition of the body that caused the discomfort. Any drug which has this deadening effect on the nerves is called a narcotic; and it is in this class that alcohol belongs, together with the stronger narcotics, opium, chloroform, ether, and chloral.

In fact, it was quickly found in the bitter school of experience that alcohol, though producing an apparent glow of warmth for the time, instead of increasing our power to resist cold, rapidly and markedly lessens it; so that those who drink heavily are much more likely to die from cold and exposure than those who let alcohol alone. Nowadays, Arctic explorers, explorers in the tropics, officers of armies upon forced marches, and those who have to train themselves for the most severe strains on their powers of endurance, all bear testimony to the fact that the use of alcohol is harmful instead of helpful under these conditions, and that it is not for a moment to be compared to real foods, like meat, sugar, or fat.

Its Effects on Working Power. Then it was claimed that alcohol increased the working power of the body; that more work and better work would be done by men at hard labor, if a little beer, or wine, was taken with their meals. Indeed, most of those who take alcohol believe that they work faster and better, and with less effort with it than without it. But the moment that this feeling of increased power and strength was submitted to careful tests in the laboratory and in the workshop, it was found that instead of more being accomplished when alcohol was taken, even in very moderate amounts, less was accomplished by from six to twelve per cent. The false sense of increased vigor and power was due to the narcotic power of alcohol to deaden the sensations of fatigue and discomfort.

It was discovered long ago, almost as soon as men began to put themselves into training for athletic feats or contests, that alcohol was not only useless, but very injurious. Any champion who, on the eve of a contest, "breaks training" by "taking a drink," knows that he is endangering his record and giving his competitors an advantage over him.

Its Deadening Effect. In short, we must conclude that the so-called stimulating effects of alcohol are really due to its power of deadening us to sensations of discomfort or fatigue. Its boasted power of making men more "sociable" by loosening their tongues is due to precisely the same effect: it takes off the balance-wheels of custom, reserve, and propriety--too often of decency, as well. This is where the greatest and most serious danger of alcohol comes in, that even in the smallest doses, it begins to deaden us both mentally and morally, and thus lessens our power of control. This loss of control steadily increases with each successive drink until finally the man, completely under the influence of liquor, reaches a stage when he can neither think rationally nor speak intelligently, nor even walk straight or stand upright--making the most humiliating and disgusting spectacle which humanity can present.

Harmful Effects on the Body. All doctors and scientists and thoughtful men are now practically agreed: First, that alcohol in excess is exceedingly dangerous and injurious, and one of the most serious enemies that modern civilization has to face.

Second, that even in the smallest doses, as a deadener of the sense of discomfort, it blinds the man who takes it to the harm it is doing and, as soon as its temporary comforting effects begin to pass off, naturally leads its victim to resort to it again in increasing doses. In fact, unlike a true food which quickly satisfies, the use of alcohol too often creates an appetite that grows by what it feeds on, and is never satisfied. For every natural appetite or instinct, nature provides a check; but she provides none for tastes that must be acquired. The last man to find out that he is taking too much is the drinker himself. Taken first to relieve discomfort, its own poisonous after-effects create a new and permanent demand for it.

The third point on which agreement is almost unanimous among scientists and physicians is that, as will be seen in later chapters, there are a considerable number of diseases of the liver, of the heart and blood vessels, of the kidneys, and of the nervous system, which are produced by, or almost always associated with, alcohol. There are, for instance, three different kinds of alcoholic insanity. It is true that these disease-changes most commonly occur in the tissues of those who use alcohol to excess; and it is also probably true that what the alcoholic poison is doing in these cases, is picking out the weak spots in the body and the weaker individuals in the community. Even the strongest and best of us have our little weaknesses of digestion, of nerves, and of disposition that we know of, as well as others that we are not acquainted with. And what is the use of running the risk of having these picked out and made worse in this dangerous and unpleasant manner, just for the sake of a little temporary indulgence?

Moreover, while it is admitted that most of these harmful effects of alcohol are produced by its use in excess, it is daily becoming a more and more difficult matter to decide just how much is "excess." It certainly differs widely in different individuals, and in different organs and parts in the same body. An amount of alcohol which one man might possibly take without harm may greatly injure another; and its frequent use, though it does not produce the slightest sign of intoxication, or even of discomfort, or headache, may be slowly and fatally damaging the cells of the liver or kidney. In fact, the conviction is growing among scientists that alcohol does the greatest harm in this slow, insidious way without its user's realizing it in any way until too late to break the fearful habit.

It may even be perfectly true that alcohol seriously injures not more than ten or fifteen per cent of those who take it in small quantities; but how can you tell whether you, or your liver, or kidney, or nerve cells, belong in the ten per cent or the ninety per cent class? On general principles, it would hardly seem worth while making the test simply for the sake of finding out. You never can quite tell what alcohol has done to you, until the post mortem (after death) examination--and then the question will not interest you very much.

Its Effect upon Character. Just as alcohol deadens the body and the senses, especially the higher ones--so it has a terrible effect upon the mental and moral sides of our natures. The results of the use of alcohol are so well known that it is unnecessary here to either describe or picture them. All that is needed is to keep our eyes open upon the street, and read the police reports. What good effects upon man's better nature has alcohol to show as an offset for this dreadful tendency to bring out the worst and lowest in man?

Increasing Knowledge of the Bad Effects of Alcohol is Decreasing its Use. It is most impressive that almost everything we have found out about alcohol in the short time that we have been studying it carefully has been to its discredit.

Fifty years ago beer and wine, all over the civilized world, were commonly regarded as foods. Now they are not considered true foods, but harmful beverages. Fifty years ago alcohol was believed to improve the digestion and increase the appetite. Now we know that it does neither. It was believed to increase working power, and has now been clearly shown to diminish it. It was supposed to increase the thinking power and stimulate the imagination, and now we know that it dulls and muddles both.

Fifty years ago it was freely used as medicine for all sorts of illnesses, both by doctor and patient; it was supposed to stimulate the heart, to sustain the strength, to increase the power of the body to resist disease, and to sustain and support life in emergencies. Now we know that practically all these claims are unfounded, and that such value as it has in medicine is chiefly as a narcotic, as a deadener of the sense of discomfort. As a result, it is already used in medicine only about one-fourth as much as it was fifty years ago, and its use is still steadily decreasing.

Fifty years ago, in this country, in England, and on the continent of Europe, farm laborers and servants living in the house, expected so many pints or quarts of ale or beer a day, as part of their regular food rations, just as they now would expect milk or tea or coffee. It was only a few years ago that the great steamship companies stopped issuing grog, or raw spirits, to the sailors in their employ, as part of their daily ration, because they at last came to realize how harmful were its effects. And a score of similar instances could be mentioned, showing that the unthinking and general use of alcohol as a beverage at our tables is steadily and constantly diminishing. Great temperance societies are springing up in this and other civilized countries and are having a powerful influence in showing the harm of the use of alcohol and in inducing people to abstain from using it.

This movement is only fairly started, but is being hastened by such practical and important influences as the experience of many of the great business corporations, such as railroads, steamship companies, insurance companies, banks, and trust companies, which support the findings of science against alcohol in almost every respect. On account of the manner in which alcohol unconsciously dulls the senses and blurs the judgment, these companies began long ago weeding out from their employ all men who were known to drink to excess; then they began to reject those who were likely to occasionally over-indulge, or take it too freely; and now, finally, many of them, particularly the railway and steamship companies, will not employ-- except in the lowest and poorest paid classes of their service--and will not promote to any position which puts men in charge of human life and limb, those who use alcohol in any form or amount.

Nearly all the captains, for instance, of our great trans-atlantic liners, whose duties in storm or fog keep them on the bridge on continuous duty for forty-eight, sixty, and even seventy-two hours at a stretch, with thousands of lives depending upon their courage and their judgment, are total abstainers. And while twenty-five years ago they used to think that they could not go through these long sieges of storm duty without plenty of wine or whiskey, they now find that they are far better off without any alcoholic drink.

Another powerful force in the same direction is our insurance companies, practically all of whom now will refuse to insure any man known habitually to use alcohol to excess, because where lists have been kept of their policy-holders showing which were users of alcohol and which total abstainers, their records show that the death rate among the users of alcohol is some twenty per cent greater than among the total abstainers. A similar result has also been reached in the companies that insure against sickness, whose drinking members average nearly twice as many weeks of sickness during the year as the abstaining ones. So both of these two great groups of business corporations are becoming powerful agencies for the promotion of temperance.

Within fifty years from now the habitual use of alcohol will probably have become quite rare. It is already becoming "good form" among the best people not to drink; and the fashion will spread, as the bad effects of alcohol become more generally understood.

TOBACCO

Smoking, a Senseless Habit. Smoking is the curious act of drawing smoke into the mouth and puffing it out again. Why this custom should have become so widespread is even a greater puzzle than is the drinking of alcohol. In civilized countries at least, it is a custom of much more recent growth than "drinking," as it was introduced into Europe from America by the early explorers, notably those sent out by Sir Walter Raleigh. As tobacco-smoke is neither a solid nor a liquid, but only a gas, no one could even pretend that it is of any value, either as food or drink. All that can be said of smoking, even by the most inveterate smoker, is that it is a habit, of no possible use or value to body or mind, and of great possibilities of harm.

Another singular thing about smoking is that its effects vary so greatly according to the individual who practices it, that scarcely any two smokers can agree as to the exact reason why they smoke, except that in some vague way smoking gives them pleasure. The only thing that they do agree upon is that they miss it greatly, and crave it keenly whenever they stop it. The only thing that stands out clearly about smoking is that while it does no good, and does not even give one definite and uniform kind of pleasure, it does form a powerful and over-mastering habit, which is exceedingly difficult to break, and develops a craving which can be satisfied only by continuing, or returning, to it.

It is Very Difficult to Break the Habit of Smoking. As a matter of practical experience, not one smoker in fifty who tries to swear off ever succeeds in doing so permanently. Why then should any one form a habit, which is of no benefit whatever, which is expensive, unpleasant to others, and which may become exceedingly injurious, simply for the sake of saddling one's self with a craving which will probably never be got rid of all the rest of one's life? The strongest and most positive thing that a smoker can say about his pipe, or cigar, or cigarette, is that he could not get along without it; and he will usually add that he wishes he had never begun to use it. You are better off in every way by letting tobacco strictly alone, and never teaching yourself to like it.

Tobacco is Not a Natural Taste. As might be expected, in the case of such an utterly useless drug, we have no natural liking or instinct for it; and the taste for it has to be acquired just as in the case of alcohol, only as a rule with greater difficulty and with more painful experiences of headache, nausea, and other discomforts.

Nicotine, a Powerful Poison. Tobacco contains and depends largely for its effects upon considerable amounts of a substance called nicotine. This is a powerful poison, even in very small doses, with only feeble narcotic, or pain-deadening, powers; but fortunately, the larger part of it is destroyed in the process of burning. Enough, however, is carried over in the smoke, or absorbed through the butt of the cigar or cigarette, or the mouth-piece of the pipe, to injure the nervous system, especially in youth. As will be seen in the chapter upon the "Care of the Heart," it especially attacks the nerves supplying the heart, and is thus most harmful to growing boys.

On account of its injurious effects upon the nerves of the heart, smoking has long been forbidden by trainers and coaches to all athletes who are training for a contest or race. In addition to its poisonous effects upon the nervous system, tobacco also does great harm to boys and young men by providing them with an attractive means of filling up their time and keeping themselves amused without either bodily or mental effort. The boy who smokes habitually will find it much easier to waste his time in day-dreams and gossip, and tends to become a loafer and an idler.

The Advantage that Non-Smokers have over Smokers. When both of these influences are taken together, it is little wonder that the investigations of Dr. Seaver, the medical director of Yale, showed that out of the 187 men in the class of 1881, those not using tobacco during their college course had gained, over the users of tobacco, twenty-two per cent in weight, twenty-nine per cent in height, nineteen per cent in growth of chest, and sixty-six per cent in increase of lung capacity.

In the Amherst graduating class for the same year, the non-users of tobacco had gained twenty-four per cent more in weight, thirty-seven per cent more in height, and forty-two per cent more in growth of chest than had the smokers. In lung capacity, the tobacco users had lost two cubic inches, while the abstainers had gained six cubic inches.

As a wet-blanket upon ambition, a drag upon development, and a handicap upon success in life, the cigarette has few equals and no superiors. The stained fingers and sallow complexion of the youthful cigarette smoker will generally result in his being rejected when applying for a position. The employer knows that the non-smoking boy is much more likely to succeed in his work and win his way to a position of trust and influence than is the "cigarette fiend." Especially in these days of sharp competition, no boy can afford to contract a habit which will so handicap him in making his way as will the cigarette habit.

CHAPTER XI

THE HEART-PUMP AND ITS PIPE-LINE SYSTEM

THE BLOOD VESSELS

Where the Body Does its Real Eating. When once the food has been dissolved in the food-tube and absorbed by the cells of its walls, the next problem is how it shall be sent all over the body to supply the different parts that are hungry for it; for we must remember that the real eating of the food is done by the billions upon billions of tiny living cells of which the body is made up.

The Pipe Lines of the Body. What do we do when we want to carry water, or oil, or sewage, quickly and surely from one place to another? We put down a pipe line. We are wonderfully proud of our systems of water and gas supply, and of the great pipe lines that carry oil from wells in Ohio and Indiana clear to the Atlantic coast. But the very first man that ever laid a pipe to carry water was simply imitating nature--only about ten or fifteen million years behind her. No sooner has our food passed through the cells in the wall of the food-tube, than it goes straight into a set of tiny tubes--the blood-pipes, or blood vessels--which carry it to the heart; and the heart pumps it all over the body.

Veins and Arteries. These blood-tubes running from the walls of the food-tube to the heart are called veins; and the other tubes through which the heart pumps the blood all over the body are called arteries. If you will spell this last word "air-teries," it may help you to remember why the name was given to these tubes ages ago. When the body was examined after death, they were found to be empty and hence were not unnaturally supposed to carry air throughout the body, and "air-teries" they have remained ever since. While absurd in one way, the name is not so far amiss in another, for an important part of their work is to carry all over the body swarms of tiny baskets, or sponges, of oxygen taken from the air.

Why the Blood is Red. The first and main purpose of the blood-pipes and the heart is to carry the dissolved food from the stomach and intestines to the cells all over the body. But the cells need air as well as food; and, to carry this, there are little basket-cells--the red corpuscles. Take a drop of blood and put it under a microscope, and you will see what they look like. The field will be simply crowded with tiny, rounded lozenges--the red cells of the blood, which give it its well-known color.

The White Corpuscles or Scavengers of the Blood. As the blood-tubes are not only supply-pipes but sewers and drainage canals as well, it is a good thing to have some kind of tiny animals living and moving about in them, which can act as scavengers and eat up some of the waste and scraps; and hence your microscope will show you another kind of little blood corpuscle, known, from the fact that it is not colored, as the white corpuscle. These corpuscles are little cells of the body, which in shape and behavior are almost exactly like an ameba--a tiny "bug," seen only under the microscope, that lives in ditch-water. Under the microscope the white corpuscles look like little round disks, about one-third larger than the red corpuscles, and with a large kernel, or nucleus, in their centre. They have the same power of changing their shape, of surrounding and swallowing scraps of food, as has the ameba, and are a combination of scavengers and sanitary police. When disease germs get into the blood, they attack and endeavor to eat and digest them; and whenever inflammation, or trouble of any sort, begins in any part of the body, they hurry to the scene in thousands, clog the blood-tubes and squeeze their way out through the walls of the smallest blood-tubes to attack the invaders or repair the damage. This causes the well-known swelling and reddening which accompanies inflammation.

Blood, then, is a sticky red fluid, two-thirds of which is food-soup, and the other third, corpuscles. How tiny the blood-corpuscles are, may be guessed from the fact that there are about 5,000,000 red cells and 10,000 white cells in every cubic centimetre (fifteen drops) of our blood.

How the Blood Circulates through the Body. Now let us see how some portion of the body, say the right thumb, gets its share of food and of oxygen through the blood. We will start at the very beginning. The food, of course, is put into the mouth, chewed by the teeth, and softened and digested in the stomach and intestines. It is then taken up by the cells of the mucous coat of the intestines and passed into the network of tiny blood-pipes surrounding them, between the lining of the bowels and their muscular coat. These tiny blood-pipes, called capillaries, run together to form larger pipes--the small veins; and the small veins from the walls of the intestine and stomach finally run together into one large pipe, or trunk-line (called the portal vein), which carries them to the liver.

In passing through the liver, the blood is purified of some irritating substances picked up from the food-tube, and the melted food which it contains is further prepared for the use of the cells of the body. The portal vein of the liver breaks up into a network of veins, and these again break up into a number of tiny capillaries, in which the blood is acted upon by the cells of the liver. These capillaries gather together again to form veins, and finally unite into two large veins at the back of the liver, which run directly into the great trunk-pipe of all the veins of the body--the vena cava (or "empty vein," so called because it is always found empty after death), about an inch from where this opens into the right side of the heart.

In the vena cava the blood from the food-tube, rich in food, but poor in oxygen, mixes with the impure, or used-up, blood brought back by the veins from all over the body and, passing into the right side of the heart, is pumped by the heart through a large blood-pipe to the lungs. This large blood-pipe divides into two branches, one for each lung; and these again break up into smaller branches, and finally into tiny capillaries, which are looped about in fine meshes, or networks, around the air-cells of the lung. Here, through the thin and delicate walls of the capillaries the blood cells give off, or breathe out, their carbon dioxid and other waste gases (which are passed out with our outgoing breath), and at the same time they breathe in oxygen which our incoming breath has drawn into the lungs.

This oxygen is picked up by, and combines with, the red coloring matter of the millions of little oxygen sponges, or baskets--the red corpuscles--and turns them a light red color, causing the blood to become bright red, such as runs in the arteries and is known as arterial blood.

The loops of tiny capillaries around the air cells of the lungs run together again to form larger pipes; and these unite, at the point of each lung nearest the heart, to form two large blood pipes--one from each lung--which pour the rich, pure blood, loaded with both food and oxygen into the left side of the heart. The left side of the heart pumps this blood out into the great main delivery-pipe for pure blood, known as the aorta, and this begins to give off branches to the different parts of the body, within a few inches of where it leaves the heart.

One of the first of these branches to be given off by the aorta is a large blood pipe, or artery, to supply the shoulder and arm; this artery runs across the chest, thence across the armpit, and down the arm to the elbow. Here it divides into two branches, one to supply the right, and the other the left, side of the forearm and hand. These branches have by this time got down to about the size of a wheat straw; the one supplying the right side is the artery which we feel throbbing in the wrist, and which we use in counting the pulse. From it run off smaller branches to supply the thumb and fingers. These branches break up again into still smaller branches, and they into a multitude of tiny capillaries, which run in every direction among all the muscle cells, delivering the food and oxygen at their very doors, as it were. The muscle cells eagerly suck out the food-stuffs, and breathe in the oxygen of the blood; at the same time, they pour into it their waste stuffs of all sorts, including carbon dioxid. These rob the blood of its bright red oxygen color and turn it a dirty purplish, or bluish, tint.

The loops of capillaries again run together, as they did in the liver and in the lung, to form tiny veins; and these run together at the base of the thumb and in the wrist, to form larger ones through which the now poor and dirty blood is carried back up the arm over much the same course as it took in coming down it. Indeed, the veins usually run parallel with, and often directly alongside of, the arteries. The blood passes through the armpit, across the chest, into the great main pipe for impure blood, the vena cava, and through this into the right side of the heart, where it again meets the rich, but waste-laden blood from the food tube and liver, and starts on its circuit through the lungs and around the body again.

The blood reaches every portion of our body in precisely this same manner, only taking a different branch of the great pure-blood delivery pipe, the aorta, according to the part of the body which it is to reach, and coming back by a different vein-pipe.

Why the Arteries are more deeply Placed than the Veins. In the limbs and over the surface of the body generally, the arteries are more deeply placed than the veins, so as to protect them from injury, because the blood in the arteries is driven at much higher pressure than in the veins and spurts out with dangerous rapidity, if they are cut. Some of the veins, indeed, run quite a little distance away from any artery and quite close to the surface of the body, so that you can see them as bluish streaks showing through the skin, particularly upon the front and inner side of the arms.

The Capillaries. Of course, the blood pipes into which the food is sucked through the walls of the food tube, and those in the lung, through which the oxygen is breathed, as well as those in the thumb through which food is taken to the muscle-cells, have the tiniest and thinnest walls imaginable. For once, the name given them by the wise men--capillaries (from the Latin capilla, a little hair)--fits them beautifully, except that the hairs in this case are hollow, and about one-twentieth of the size of the finest hair you can see with the naked eye. So tiny are they that they compare with the big veins near the heart into which they finally empty much as the smallest and slenderest twigs of an elm do with its trunk. What they lack in size, however, they more than make up in numbers; and a network of them as fine and close as the most delicate gauze goes completely around the food tube between its mucous lining and muscular coat.

Though thickest and most abundant on the inner and outer surfaces of the body, every particle of the body substance is shot through and through with a network of these tiny tubes. So close and fine is this network in the skin, for instance, that, as you can readily prove, it is impossible to thrust the point of the finest needle through the skin without piercing one of them and "drawing blood," as we say, or making it bleed. From this network of tiny, thin-walled tubes, the body-cells draw their food from the blood.

The Meaning of Good Color. It is the red blood in this spongy network of tiny vessels that gives a pink coloring to our lips and the flush of health to our cheeks. Whenever for any reason the blood is less richly supplied with food or oxygen, or more loaded with "smoke" and other body dirt than it should be, we lose this good color and become pale or sallow. If we will remember that our hearts, our livers, our brains, and our stomachs, are at the same time often equally "pale" and sallow--that is, badly supplied with blood--as our complexions, we can readily understand why it is that we are likely to have poor appetites, poor memories, bad tastes in our mouths, and are easily tired whenever, as we say, our "blood is out of order." The blood is the life. Starve or poison that, and you starve or poison every bit of living stuff in the body.

THE HEART

Structure and Action of the Heart. Now what is it that keeps the blood whirling round and round the body in this wonderful way? It is done by a central pump (or more correctly, a little explosive engine), with thick muscular walls, called the heart, which every one knows how to find by putting the hand upon the left side of the chest and feeling it beat. The heart is really a bulb, or pouch, which has ballooned out from the central feed pipe of the blood supply system, somewhat in the same way that the stomach has ballooned out from the food tube.

The walls of this pouch, or bulb, are formed of a thick layer of very elastic and powerful muscles almost as thick as the palm of your hand. When the great vein trunk has poured blood into this pouch until it is swollen full and tight, these muscles in its walls shut down sharply and squirt or squeeze the blood in the heart-pouch into the great artery-pipe, the aorta. In fact, you can get a very fair, but rough, idea of the way in which the heart acts by putting your half-closed hand down into a bowl of water and then suddenly squeezing it till it is shut tight, driving the water out of the hollow of your hand in a jet, or squirt.

"But," some of you will ask at once, "what is to prevent the blood in the heart, when the muscle wall squeezes down upon it, from shooting backward into the vena cava, instead of forward into the aorta?"

Nature thought of that long ago, and ingeniously but very simply guarded against it by causing two little folds of the lining of the blood pipes to stick up both where the vena cava enters the heart and where the aorta leaves it, so as to form little flaps which act as valves. These valves allow the blood to flow forward, but snap together and close the opening as soon as it tries to flow backward. While largest and best developed in the heart, these valves are found at intervals of an inch or two all through the veins in most parts of the body, allowing the blood to flow freely toward the heart, but preventing it from flowing back.

As the heart has to pump all the blood in the body twice,--once around and through the lungs, and once around and through the whole of the body,--it has become divided into two halves, a right half, which pumps the blood through the lungs and is slightly the smaller and the thinner walled of the two; and a left half, which pumps the purified blood, after it has come back from the lungs, all over the rest of the body.

Each half, or side, of the heart has again divided itself into a receiving cavity, or pouch, known as the auricle; and a pumping or delivering pouch, known as the ventricle. And another set of valves has grown up between the auricle and the ventricle on each side of the heart. These valves have become very strong and tough, and are tied back in a curious and ingenious manner by tough little guy ropes of tendon, or fibrous tissues, such as you can see quite plainly in the heart of an ox. It is important for you to remember this much about them, because, as we shall see in the next chapter, these valves are one of the parts of the heart most likely to wear out, or become diseased.

Heart Beat and Pulse. The heart fills and empties itself about eighty times a minute, varying from one hundred and twenty times for a baby, and ninety for a child of seven, to eighty for a woman, and seventy-two for a full-grown man.

When the walls of the ventricles squeeze down to drive out their blood into the lungs and around the body, like all other muscles they harden as they contract and thump the pointed lower end, or apex, of the heart against the wall of the chest, thus making what is known as the beat of the heart, which you can readily feel by laying your hand upon the left side of your chest, especially after you have been running or going quickly upstairs. As each time the heart beats, it throws out half a teacupful of blood into the aorta, this jet sends a wave of swelling down the arteries all over the body, which can be felt clearly as far away as the small arteries of the wrist and the ankle. This wave of swelling, which, of course, occurs as often as the heart beats, is called the pulse; and we "take" it, or count and feel its force and fullness, to estimate how fast the heart is beating and how well it is doing its work. We generally use an artery in the wrist (radial) for this purpose because it is one of the largest arteries in the body which run close to the surface and can be easily reached.

Summary of the Circulation of the Blood. We will now sum up, and put together in their order, the different things we have learned about the circulation of the blood through the body.

Starting from the great vein trunk, the vena cava, it pours into the receiving chamber, or auricle, of the right side of the heart, passes between the valves of the opening into the lower chamber, the right ventricle. When this is full, the muscles in the wall of the ventricle contract, the valve flaps fly up, and the blood is squirted out through the pulmonary artery to the lungs. Here it passes through the capillaries round the air cells, loses its carbon dioxid, takes in oxygen, and is gathered up and returned through great return pipes to the receiving chamber, or auricle, of the left side of the heart. Here it collects while the ventricle below is emptying itself, then pours down between the valve flaps through the opening to the left ventricle. When this is full, it contracts; the valves fly up and close the orifice; and the blood is squirted out through another valve-guarded opening, into the great main artery, the aorta. This carries it, through its different branches, all over the body, where the tissues suck out their food and oxygen through the walls of the capillaries, and return it through the small veins into the large vein pipes, which again deliver it into the vena cava, and so to the right side of the heart from which we started to trace it.

Although the two sides of the heart are doing different work, they contract and empty themselves, and relax and fill themselves, at the same time, so that we feel only one beat of the whole heart.

One of the most wonderful things about the entire system of blood tubes is the way in which each particular part and organ of the body is supplied with exactly the amount of blood it needs. If the whole body is put to work, so that a quicker circulation of blood, with its millions of little baskets of oxygen, is needed to enable the tissues to breathe faster, the heart meets the situation by beating faster and harder. This, as you all know, you can readily cause by running, or jumping, or wrestling.

CHAPTER XII

THE CARE OF THE HEART-PUMP AND ITS PIPE-LINES

The Effect of Work upon the Heart. Whatever else in this body of ours may be able to take a rest at times, the heart never can. When it stops, we stop! Naturally, with such a constant strain upon it, we should expect it to have a tendency to give way, or break down, at certain points. The real wonder is that it breaks down so seldom. It has great powers of endurance and a wonderful trick of patching up break-downs and adjusting itself to strains.

Every kind of work, of course, done in the body throws more work upon the heart. When we run, or saw wood, our muscles contract, and need more food-fuel to burn, and pour more waste-stuff into the blood to be thrown off through the lungs; so the heart has to beat harder and faster to supply these calls. When our stomach digests food, it needs a larger supply of blood in its walls, and the heart has to pump harder to deliver this. Even when we think hard or worry over something, our brain cells need more blood, and the ever-willing heart again pumps it up to them. This is the chief reason why we cannot do more than one of these things at a time to advantage. If we try to think hard, run foot races, and digest our dinner all at one and the same time, neither head, stomach, nor muscles can get the proper amount of blood that it requires; we cannot do any one of the three properly, and are likely to develop a headache, or an attack of indigestion, or a "stitch in the side," and sometimes all three. So the circulation has a great deal to do with the intelligent planning and arranging of our work, our meals, and our play. If we are going to increase our endurance, we must increase the power of our heart and blood vessels, as well as that of our muscles. The real thing to be trained in the gymnasium and on the athletic field is the heart rather than the muscles.

Fortunately, however, the heart is itself a muscle, alive and growing, and with the same power of increasing in strength and size that any other muscle has. So that up to a proper limit, all these things which throw strain upon the heart in moderate degree, such as running, working, and thinking, are not only not harmful, but beneficial to it, increasing both its strength and its size. The heart, for instance, of a thoroughbred race-horse is nearly twice the size, in proportion to his body weight, of the heart of a dray-horse or cart-horse; and a deer has more than twice as large a heart as a sheep of the same weight.

The important thing to bear in mind in both work and play, in athletic training, and in life, is that this work must be kept easily within the powers of the heart and of the other muscles, and must be increased gradually, and never allowed to go beyond a certain point, or it becomes injurious, instead of beneficial; hurtful, instead of helpful. Over-work in the shop or factory, overtraining in the gymnasium or on the athletic field, both fall first and heaviest upon the heart.

Importance of Food, Air, and Exercise. At the same time, the system must be kept well supplied through the stomach with the raw material both for doing this work and for building up this new muscle. When anyone, in training for an event, gets "stale," or overtrained, and loses his appetite and his sleep, he had better stop at once, for that is a sign that he is using more energy than his food is able to give him through his stomach; and the stomach has consequently "gone on a strike."

How to Avoid Heart Overstrain and Heart Disease. The way, then, to avoid overstrain and diseases of the heart and blood vessels is:--

First, to take plenty of exercise, but to keep that exercise within reasonable limits, which, in childhood, ought to be determined by a school physician, and in workshops and factories by a state factory physician.

Second, to take that exercise chiefly in the open air, and as much of it as possible in the form of play, so that you can stop whenever you begin to feel tired or your heart throbs too hard--in other words, whenever nature warns you that you are approaching the danger line.

Third, to keep yourself well supplied with plenty of nutritious, wholesome, digestible food, so as to give yourself, not merely power to do the work, but something besides to grow on.

Fourth, to avoid poisonous and hurtful things like the toxins of infectious diseases; and alcohol, tobacco, and other narcotics, which have a harmful effect upon the muscles, valves, or nerves of your heart, or the walls of your blood vessels.

Fortunately, the heart is so wonderfully tough and elastic, and can repair itself so rapidly, that it usually takes at least two, and sometimes three, causes acting together, to produce serious disease or damage. For instance, while muscular overwork and overstrain alone may cause serious and even permanent damage to the heart, they most frequently do so in those who are underfed, or badly housed, or recovering from the attack of some infectious disease. While the poisons of rheumatism and alcohol will alone cause serious damage to the valves of the heart and walls of the blood vessels, yet they again are much more liable to do so in those who are overworked, or underfed, or overcrowded.

The Disease of the Stiffening of the Arteries. The points at which our pipe-line system is most likely to give way are the valves of the heart, and, more likely still, the muscles of the heart wall and of the walls of the blood vessels. These little muscles are slowly, but steadily, changing all through life, becoming stiffer and less elastic, less alive, in fact, until finally, in old age, they become stiff and rigid, turning into leathery, fibrous tissue, and may even become so soaked with lime salts as to become brittle, so that they may burst under some sudden strain. When this occurs in one of the arteries of the brain, it causes an attack of apoplexy, or a "stroke of paralysis." Overstrain, or toxins in the blood, may bring about this stiffening of the arteries too soon, and then, we say that the person is "old before his time." A man is literally "as old as his arteries."

The causes which will hasten the stiffening of the arteries are, first of all, prolonged overwork and overstrain,--due especially to long hours of steady work in unwholesome shops or surroundings; second, the presence in the blood of the poisons of the more chronic infectious diseases, like tuberculosis; third, the waste products that are formed in our own body, and are not properly got rid of through lungs, skin, and kidneys; and fourth, the use of alcohol, tobacco, and other narcotics.

The Bad Effects of Alcohol. Alcohol is particularly likely to damage the walls of the blood vessels and the heart, first, because it is a direct poison to their cells, when taken in excess, and often in what may appear to be moderate amounts, if long continued; secondly, because it is frequently taken, especially by the poorer, underfed class of workers, as a substitute for food, causing them literally to "spend their money for that which is not bread," and to leave their tissues half-starved; and thirdly, because, by its narcotic effects, it decreases respiration and clogs the kidneys and the skin, thus preventing the waste products from leaving the body.

How the Heart Valves may be Injured. The valves of the heart are likely to give way, partly because they are under such constant strain, snapping backward and forward day and night; and partly, because, in order to be thin enough and strong enough for this kind of work, they have become turned, almost entirely, into stringy, half-dead, fibrous tissue, which has neither the vitality nor the resisting power of the live body-stuffs like muscles, gland-cells, and nerves. They are so tough, however, that they seldom give way under ordinary wear and tear, as the leather of a pump valve, or of your shoes, might; but the thing which damages them, nine times out of ten, is the germs or poisons of some infectious disease.

These poisons circulating through the blood, sometimes set up a severe inflammation in the valves and the lining of the heart. Ulcers, or little wart-like growths, form on the valves; and these may either eat away and destroy entirely parts of the valves or, when they heal, leave scars which shorten and twist the valves out of shape, so that they can no longer close the openings. When this has happened, the heart is in the condition of a pump which will not hold water, because the leather valve in its bucket is broken or warped; and we say that the patient has valvular or organic heart disease.

The disease which most frequently causes this serious defect is rheumatism, or rheumatic fever; but it may also occur after pneumonia, typhoid, blood poisoning, or even after a common cold, or an attack of the grip. This is one of several reasons why we should endeavor, in every way, to avoid and stop the spread of these infectious diseases; not only are they dangerous in themselves, but although only two of them, rheumatism and pneumonia, frequently attack the heart, all of them do so occasionally, and together they cause nearly nine-tenths of all cases of organic heart disease.

Should you be unfortunate enough to catch one of these diseases, the best preventive against its attacking the heart, or causing serious damage, if it does, is a very simple one--rest in bed until the fever is all gone and your doctor says it is perfectly safe for you to get up; and avoid any severe muscular strain for several months afterward.

This is a most important thing to remember after all infections and fevers, no matter how mild. Even where the heart valves have been seriously attacked, as in rheumatism, they will often recover almost completely if you keep at rest, and your heart is not overtaxed by the strain of heavy, muscular work, before it has entirely recovered. Ten days' "taking it easy" after a severe cold, or a bad sore throat, may save you a serious strain upon the heart, from which you might be months or even years in recovering.

But even where serious damage has been done to the heart, so that one of its valves leaks badly, nature is not at the end of her resources. She simply sets to work to build up and strengthen and thicken the heart muscle until it is strong enough to overcome the defect and pump blood enough to keep the body properly supplied--just as, if you are working with a leaky pump, you will have to pump harder and faster in order to keep a good stream of water flowing. It is astonishing how completely she will make good the loss of even a considerable part of a valve.

Doctors no longer forbid patients with heart disease to take exercise, but set them at carefully planned exercise in the open air, particularly walking and hill-climbing; at the same time feeding them well, so as to assist nature in building up and strengthening the heart muscle until it can overcome the defect. In this way, they may live, with reasonable care, ten, fifteen, or twenty years--often, in fact, until they die of something else.

Don't worry about your heart if it should happen to palpitate, or take a "hop-skip-and-jump" occasionally. You will never get real heart disease until you have had some fever or serious illness, which leaves you short of breath for a long time afterward.

Danger to the Heart through the Nervous System. The other chief way in which the heart may be affected is through the nervous system. Being the great supply pump for the entire body, it is, of course, connected most thoroughly and elaborately by nerve wires with the brain and, through it, with every other organ in the body. So delicately is it geared,--set on such a hair-trigger, as it were,--that it not only beats faster when work is done anywhere in the body, but begins to hurry in anticipation of work to be done anywhere. You all know how your heart throbs and beats like a hammer and goes pit-a-pat when you are just expecting to do something important,--for instance, to speak a piece or strike a fast ball,--or even when you are greatly excited watching somebody else do something, as in the finish of a close race.

Two-thirds of the starts and jumps and throbbings that the heart makes, are due to excitement, or nervous overstrain, or the fact that your dinner is not digesting properly; and they don't indicate anything serious at all, but are simply useful danger signals to you that something is not just right.

In work and in athletics for instance, this rapid and uncomfortably vigorous action of the heart is one of nature's best checks and guides. When your heart begins to throb and plunge uncomfortably, you should slow up until it begins to quiet down again, and you will seldom get into serious trouble. The next time you try the same feat, you will probably find that you can go a little farther, or faster, without making it throb. Indeed, getting into training is very largely getting the heart built up and educated, so that you can run or play, or wrestle hard without overtaxing it. Whatever you can do within the limits of your heart is safe, wholesome, and invigorating; whatever goes beyond this, is dangerous and likely to be injurious.

Occasionally, however, some of the nerves which control the heart become disturbed or diseased so that, instead of the heart's simply beating harder and faster whenever more blood is really needed, it either throbs and beats a great deal harder and faster than is necessary, or goes racing away on its own account, and beats "for dear life," when there is no occasion for it, thus tiring itself out without doing any good, and producing a very unpleasant feeling of nervousness and discomfort. This may be due to overwork, whether with muscles or brain; or to worry or loss of sleep, in which case it means that you must put on the brakes, take plenty of rest and exercise in the open air, and get plenty of sleep. Then these danger signals, having accomplished their warning purpose, will disappear.

Other Causes of Heart Trouble. At other times, this palpitation is due to the presence of poisons in the blood, either those of infectious disease, or of certain waste products produced in the body in excess, as, for instance, when your digestion is out of order, or your skin, kidneys, and bowels are not working properly; or it is due to tea, coffee, or tobacco.

Effects of Tea and Coffee. Tea and coffee, if taken in excess, will sometimes produce very uncomfortable palpitation, or rapid over-action of the heart, with restlessness and inability to sleep. They usually act in this way only when taken in large amounts, or upon a small percentage of persons who are peculiarly affected by them; and this palpitation is seldom serious, and disappears when their excessive use is stopped.

Tobacco and its Dangers to the Heart. Tobacco has a very injurious effect upon the nerves of the heart in the young, making them so irritable that the heart will beat very rapidly on the least exertion; so that gradually one becomes less and less inclined to attempt exertion of any sort, whether bodily or mental, and falls into a stagnant, stupid sort of condition which seriously interferes with both growth and progress.

In other cases, tobacco dulls and deadens the nerves controlling the heart, as it does the rest of the nervous system and the brain, so that the smoker feels as if nothing were worth while doing very hard, and it becomes difficult for him to fix his mind upon a subject. At the same time, it dulls the appetite so that one takes less wholesome food; and it checks, or clogs up, the sewer-pipes of the skin, the liver, and the kidneys.

Of course, as you know, all trainers and coaches, even though they be habitual smokers themselves, absolutely forbid tobacco in any form to athletes who are training for a contest, on account of its effects upon the nervous system and the heart.

A certain percentage of individuals are peculiarly susceptible to tobacco, so that it has a special poisonous effect upon the nerves of the heart, causing a rapid pulse and shortness of breath, known as tobacco heart. This is not of very common occurrence; but it is exceedingly troublesome when it does occur, and it takes a long time to get over it, even after the use of tobacco has been stopped entirely. Sometimes it leads to permanent damage of the nerves and of the heart.

Give your heart plenty of vigorous exercise, but don't make it beat uncomfortably hard. Give it plenty of food, sleep, and fresh air; avoid poisoning it, either with the toxins of diseases, or with your own waste-poisons, or alcohol, or tobacco; and it will serve you faithfully till a good old age.

CHAPTER XIII

HOW AND WHY WE BREATHE

Life is Shown by Breathing. If you wanted to find out whether a little black bunch up in the branches of a tree were a bird or a cluster of leaves, or a brown blur in the stubble were a rabbit or a clod, the first thing you would probably look for would be to see whether it moved, and secondly, if you could get close enough without its moving away, whether it were breathing. You would know perfectly well if you saw it breathing that it was alive, and that, if it were not breathing at all, it would probably be dead, or very nearly so.

Why is breathing so necessary to life that it lasts practically as long as life does, and when it stops, life stops too? Animals can stop eating for days, or even weeks, and yet live, especially if they were fairly fat when they began to fast. Indeed, some animals, like woodchucks, bears, and marmots, will go to sleep in the fall, and sleep right on through to spring without eating a mouthful. But if any animal or bird is prevented from breathing for three minutes, it will die.

Short Storage Supply of Air. There is a difference between the kind of things that you take in when you breathe and the kind of things you take in when you eat or drink. Food and drink are solids and liquids; and the body is a great sponge of one soaked full of the other, so that large amounts of food and water can be stored up in the body. But what you take in when you breathe is, of course, air--which is neither a solid nor a liquid, but a gas, very light and bulky. Of gases the body can soak up and hold only a very small amount; so its storage supply of them will be used up completely in about three minutes, and then it dies if it cannot get more air.

Why our Bodies Need Air-Oxidation. The body is made up of millions of tiny living animals called cells, which eat the food that is brought to them from the blood and pour their waste and dirt back again into the same current. Now, what would happen if we were to throw all the garbage from the kitchen, and the wash water from the kitchen sink, and the dirty water from the bathroom right into the well out of which we pumped our drinking water? We should simply be poisoned within two or three days, if indeed we could manage to drink the disgusting mixture at all. That is exactly what would happen to our body cells if they were not provided with some way of getting rid of their waste and dirt.

Part of the waste that comes from our body cells is either watery, or easily dissolved in water; and this is carried in the blood to a special set of filter organs--the liver and the kidneys--and poured out of the body as the urine. Another part of it, when circulating through the skin, is passed off in the form of that watery vapor which we call perspiration, or sweat. But part of the waste can be got rid of only by burning, and what we call burning is another name for combining with oxygen, or to use one word--oxidation; and this is precisely the purpose of the carrying of oxygen by the little red blood cells from the lungs to the deeper parts of the body--to burn up, or oxidize, these waste materials which would otherwise poison our cells. When they are burnt, or oxidized, they become almost harmless.

Why the Red Cells Carry only Oxygen to the Body. But why do not the red cells carry air instead of just oxygen? This is simply a clever little economy of space on nature's part. As a chemist will tell you the air which we breathe is a mixture of two gases--one called nitrogen and the other oxygen; just as syrup, for instance, is a mixture of sugar and water. Then too, as in syrup, there are different amounts of the two substances in the mixture: as syrup is made up of about one-quarter sugar and three-quarters water, so air is made up of one-fifth oxygen and four-fifths nitrogen. Now the interesting thing about this mixture, which we call air, is that the only really "live" and vital part of it for breathing purposes is the one-fifth of oxygen, the four-fifths of nitrogen being of no use to our lungs. In fact, if you split up the air with an electric current, or by some other means, and thus divide it into a small portion of pure oxygen (one-fifth), and a very much larger portion (four-fifths) of nitrogen, the latter would as promptly suffocate the animal that tried to breathe it as if he were plunged under water.[18]

It may perhaps be difficult to think of anything burning inside of your bodies where everything is moist, especially as you do not see any flame; but you do find there one thing which always goes with burning, and that is warmth, or heat. This slow but steady and never-ceasing burning, or oxidation, of the waste and dirt inside your bodies is what keeps them warm. When you run fast, or wrestle, or work hard, your muscle-cells work faster, and make more waste, and you breathe faster to get in the oxygen to burn this up--in other words, you fan the body fires, and in consequence you get a great deal hotter, and perhaps perspire in order to get rid of your surplus heat.

The Ocean of Air. Where does the blood in the body go in order to get this oxygen, which is so vital to it? Naturally, somewhere upon the surface of the body, because we are surrounded by air wherever we sit, or stand, or move, just as fishes are by water. All outdoors, as we say, is full of air. We are walking, just as fishes swim, at the bottom of an ocean of air some thirty miles deep; and the nearer we get up toward the surface of that ocean, as, for instance, when we climb a high mountain, the lighter and thinner the air becomes. Above ten thousand feet we often have great difficulty in breathing properly, because the air is so thin and weak in oxygen.

How the Lungs Grew Up. In the simplest forms of life, any part of the soft and delicate surface will do for the blood to reach, in order to throw off its load of carbon "smoke" and take on its supply of oxygen. In fact, animals like jellyfish and worms are lungs all over. But as bodies begin to get bigger, and the skin begins to toughen and harden, this becomes more and more difficult, although even the highest and biggest animals like ourselves still throw off a certain amount of this carbon dioxid and other gases through the skin. Accordingly, certain parts of the surface of the body are set apart specially for this business of breathing; and as we already have an opening into the body provided by the mouth and food tube, the simplest thing to do is to use the mouth for taking in air, when it is not being used for taking in food, and to set aside some part of the food tube for breathing purposes.

The lungs sprout out from the front of the gullet, just below the root of the tongue, in the days when we are getting ready to be born. The sprout divides into two, forming the beginning of the pair of lungs. Each lung sprout again divides into two, and each of the two smaller buds again into two, until finally we have the whole chest filled up with a "lung-tree" whose trunk stems and leaves are hollow. The stem of the tree or bush becomes the windpipe (trachea). The first two branches into which it divides form the right and left lung tubes, known as bronchi. The third, fourth, fifth, sixth, etc., divisions, and so on, form what are known as the bronchial tubes. These keep on splitting into tinier and tinier twigs, until they end, like the bush, in little leaves, which in the lung, of course, are hollow and are called the air cells (alveoli). This budding off of the lungs from the gullet is the reason why the air we breathe and the food we swallow go down the same passage. Every mouthful of our food slides right across the opening of the windpipe, which has to be protected by a special flap, or trap-door of gristle, called the epiglottis. If you try to eat and talk at the same time, the epiglottis doesn't get warning of the coming of a swallow of food in time to cover the opening of the windpipe, and the food goes down the wrong way and you cough and choke.

Now, if you will just place your fingers upon the front of your neck and slide them up and down, you will, at once, feel your windpipe--a hard, rounded tube with ridges running across it,--while, no matter how carefully you feel, or how deeply you press, you cannot feel your gullet or esophagus at all. Just take a mouthful of water, however, put your fingers deeply on each side of the windpipe, and swallow, and you will feel something shoot down the esophagus, between your fingers, toward the stomach.

Both of these tubes were made of exactly the same materials to begin with. Why have they become so different? A moment's thought will tell you. One, the gullet, has only to swallow solid food or drink, so that its walls can remain soft, and indeed fall together, except when it is actually swallowing. The other tube, the air-pipe or windpipe, has to carry air, which neither will fall of its own weight, nor can readily be gulped down or belched up. It is absolutely necessary that its walls should become stiff enough to keep it open constantly and let the air flow backward and forward. So we find growing up in the walls of this air pipe, cells which turn themselves into rings of gristle, or cartilage.

What the Breath Is. As you know, your "breath," as you call it,--that is to say, the used-up air which you blow out of your lungs,--is different in several ways from pure, or unused air. In the first place, it is likely to have a slight musky or mousy odor about it. You never like to breathe any one else's breath, or have any one breathe in your face. This dislike is due to certain gases, consisting of impurities from the blood, the cells of the lungs, the throat, the nose, and, if the mouth is open, the teeth. These are not only offensive and disagreeable to smell, but poisonous to breathe.

Then your breath is much warmer than the rest of the air. In fact, on a very cold morning you may have tried to warm up your fingers by breathing on them; and you have also noticed that if a number of people are shut up in a room with doors and windows closed, it soon begins to feel hot as well as stuffy. This heat, of course, is given off from the blood in the lungs and in the walls of the throat and nose, as the air passes in and out again.

When you stand at the window on a cold day, the glass just in front of your mouth clouds over, so that you can no longer see through it; and if you rub your finger across this cloud, it comes away wet. Evidently, the air is moister than it was when you breathed it in; this moisture also has been given off from the blood in the lungs.

But what of the principal waste gas that the blood gives off in the lungs--the carbon "smoke," or carbon dioxid? Can you see any trace of this in the breath? No, you cannot, for the reason that this gas is like air, perfectly clear and transparent, and never turns to moisture at any ordinary temperature. But it has a power of combining with certain other things and forming substances which, because they are combinations of carbon, are called carbonates. The commonest substance with which it will do this is lime. If you take a glass or a bottle two-thirds full of lime water, and breathe into it through a glass tube or straw, you will see in a very few minutes that it is becoming milky or cloudy from the formation of visible carbonate of lime, which, when you get enough of it, makes ordinary limestone. So, although you cannot see, or smell, this carbon "smoke" in your breath, you can readily prove that it is present.

How and Why our Breathing Varies. When you run or wrestle, you breathe faster in order to draw more air into the lungs. At the same time, your heart beats faster in order to drive a larger amount of blood through the lungs. If you run too far, or wrestle too hard, your heart and your lungs both go faster and faster, until finally they reach a point when they cannot go any quicker, and the poisonous waste substances are formed in your muscles faster than they can possibly be burned up, even by the quickest breathing and the hardest pumping of your heart. Then you begin to get "out of breath"; and if you were compelled--in order to save your life, for instance--to keep on running, or fighting, you would at last be suffocated by your own waste and dirt, and fall exhausted, or unconscious.

On the other hand, by carefully training your muscles and your heart and your lungs by exercises of various sorts in the open air, beginning with easy ones and going on to harder and longer ones, you can "improve your wind," so that your heart will be able to pump more blood through the lungs per minute, and your lungs will be able to expand themselves more fully and more rapidly without fatigue.

If you can recall having had a fever of any sort, even a slight one, such as comes with a sore throat or a bad cold, you may remember that you breathed faster and that your heart beat faster, and yet you were not doing any work with your muscles. The cause, however, is the same; namely, the amount of waste that is being produced in the body--in this case, by the poisons (toxins) of the germs that cause the fever. The more waste that is formed in the body, the more effort the heart and lungs will make to try to get rid of it.

The Ribs. How does the air get in and out of the lung tubes? Evidently you do not and cannot swallow it as you would food or drink; and as it will not run down of its own accord when you simply open your mouth, nature has had to devise a special bit of machinery for the purpose of sucking it in and pressing it out again. This she has done in a rather ingenious manner by causing certain of the muscle-rings in the wall of the chest to turn first into gristle, or cartilage, and then later into bone, making what are known as the ribs; these run round the chest much as hoops do round a barrel, or as the whalebone rings did in the old-fashioned hoop skirt. When the muscles of the chest pull these ribs up, the chest is made larger,--like a bellows when you lift the handle,--air is sucked in, and we "breathe in" as we say; when the muscles let go, the ribs sink, the chest flattens and becomes smaller, the air is driven out, and we "breathe out."

FOOTNOTES:

[18] This nitrogen, though of no value for breathing, is of great value as a food, forming, as we have seen, an important part of all meats, or proteins, which build the tissues of our bodies. It can, however, be taken from the air only with great difficulty, by a very roundabout route; the bacteria of the soil eat it first, then they pass it on as food to the roots of plants; animals eat plants, and we eat the animals, and thus get most of our nitrogen.

CHAPTER XIV

HOW TO KEEP THE LUNG-BELLOWS IN GOOD CONDITION

THE NEED OF PURE AIR

Free Air is Pure. As air, in the form of wind, actually sweeps all outdoors, day and night, it clearly is likely to pick up a good many different kinds of dust and dirt, which may not be wholesome when breathed into our lungs. Fortunately, nature's great outdoor system of purifying the air is almost perfect, so that it is only when we build houses and shut in air from the great outdoor circulation, that "dirt" that is really dangerous begins to get into it. Caged air is the only air that is dangerous. Free-moving air is always perfectly safe to breathe any hour of the day or night, or any season of the year.

Shut-in and Stagnant Air is Foul. This restless air-gas cannot be stored outside of the body, any better than it can be inside. For one thing, it is too bulky; and for another, it begins to become impure in various ways, as soon as it is shut up. It is the most unmanageable food that we "eat," for we can neither cook it nor wash it like solid food, nor filter it nor boil it like water, except on a very limited scale. We can do nothing to it except to foul it, which we do with every breath that we breathe, every fire that we make, every factory that we build. Our only chance of safety, our only hope of life, is to connect every room and every corner of those little brick and mortar boxes, those caged sections of out-of-doors, that we call houses, with nature's great system of air supply, "All Outdoors." Fortunately, the only thing needed to make the connection is to open a window--no need to send for a plumber or put in a meter, and there is no charge for the supply after connections have been made.

The Enormous Amount of Air. Air outdoors is everywhere, for practical purposes, absolutely pure, just as water is when it comes down from the clouds. And like water, its only dangerous impurities are what we put there ourselves. The purity of outdoor air is due mainly to the fact that there is such an enormous amount of it, not only the miles and miles of it that stretch away on every side of us, but nearly thirty miles of it straight up above our heads; its purity is also due to the fact that, like water, it is always in motion. When heated by the sun, it expands; and, in doing so, it rises because it is less dense and therefore lighter. As soon as the pressure of the air above is lessened, air rushes in below from all the cooler regions around. This rushing of air we call a wind. If the low pressure lies to the north of us, the air rushes northward over us to fill it, and we say the wind is from the south; if the air is flowing to the south of us, we say the wind is from the north.

How Air is Purified. In these winds certain small amounts of dust, or dirt, or leaf mould are whirled up into the air, but these are promptly washed down again whenever it rains; and the same is true of the smoke impurities in the air of our great cities. Air is also constantly being purified by the heat and light of the sunbeams, burned clean in streaks by the jagged bolt of the lightning in summer, and frozen sweet and pure by the frosts every winter. So that air in the open, or connected with the open, and free to move as it will, is always pure and wholesome. But to be sure of this, it must be "eaten alive"-- that is, in motion. Stagnant air is always dead and, like all dead things, has begun to decay.

The Carbon Dioxid in the Air. Air, as you will remember (p. 132), is a mixture of oxygen and nitrogen, and its value in the body is that it gives off part of its oxygen to combine with the body wastes and burn them to carbon dioxid. Oddly enough, even pure outdoor air contains tiny traces of carbon dioxid; but the amount is so very small as to be of no practical importance, in spite of the fact that every kind of animal that lives and moves upon the earth is pouring it out from his lungs every second. The rapidity with which it disappears is due in part to the rapidity with which it rises and spreads, or is blown, in every direction; and in part to the wonderful arrangement by which, while animals throw off this poisonous gas as waste, plants eagerly suck it in through the pores in their leaves and eat it, turning it into the carbohydrates, starch and sugar, which, in turn, become valuable foods for the animals. So perfect is this system of escape, or blowing away, of carbon dioxid, combined with its being eaten up by plants, that even the air over our great cities and manufacturing towns contains only the merest trifle more of carbon dioxid than that over the open country. Its other smoke-impurities, dirts and dusts, escape, or are blown away so rapidly that they are seldom thick enough to be injurious to health, except in the narrowest and darkest streets; so that it is always safe to open your windows wide for air, wherever you may live. The principal danger from smoke is that it cuts off the sunlight.

The Necessity for Ventilation--Impurities of Indoor Air. The worst impurities in air are those that come from our own breaths and our own bodies; and, unexpectedly enough, carbon dioxid is not one of them. In spite of hundreds of experiments, we do not yet know exactly what these impurities are, though they are doubtless given off from our lungs, our skins, our mouths, and teeth, especially if the latter are not kept clean and sweet, but left dirty and decaying.

We do know, however, to a certainty that air shut up in a room, or house, with people, rapidly becomes poisonous and unwholesome. As we breathe on an average about eighteen or twenty times to the minute when we are grown up, and twenty-five to thirty times a minute when we are children, you can readily see how quickly the air in an ordinary-sized room will be used up, and how foul and unfit for further breathing it will become from being loaded with these bad-smelling lighter gases, with the carbon "smoke," with heat, and with moisture. The only way in which a room can be kept fit for human beings to breathe in is to have a draught, or current of air, pouring into it through open windows, or open doors, or ventilating shafts, at least as rapidly as it is being breathed by the persons who occupy that room. By hundreds of tests this has now been found to be on an average about four bushels a minute for each person, and any system of proper ventilation must supply this amount of air in order to make a room fit to sit in.

If a man, for instance, accidentally gets shut into a bank-vault, or other air-tight box or chamber, it will be only a few minutes before he begins to feel suffocated; and in a few hours he will be dead, unless some one opens the door. A century ago, when the voyage from Europe to America was made in sailing vessels, whenever a violent storm came up, in the smaller and poorer ships the hatches were closed and nailed down to keep the great waves which swept over the decks from pouring down the cabin-stairs and swamping the ship. If they were kept closed for more than two days, it was no uncommon thing to find two or three children or invalids among the unfortunate emigrants dead of slow suffocation; and many of those who were alive would later have pneumonia and other inflammations of the lungs. On one or two horrible occasions, when the crew had had a hard fight to save the ship and were afraid to open the hatches even for a moment, nearly one-third of the passengers were found dead when the storm subsided. So it is well to remember that we are fearfully poisonous to ourselves, unless we give nature full chance to ventilate us.

There are also other ways in which the air in houses may be made impure besides by our own bodies, but none of them is half so serious or important. All the lights that we burn in a house, except electric ones, are eating up oxygen and giving off carbon dioxid. In fact, a burning gas jet will do almost as much toward fouling the air of a room as a grown man or woman, and should be counted as a person when arranging for ventilation.

If gas pipes should leak, so that the gas escapes into a room, it is very injurious and unwholesome--indeed, in sufficient amounts, it will suffocate. Or, if the sewer pipes in the walls of the house, or in the ground under the cellar, are not properly trapped and guarded, sewer gas may escape into the house from them, and this also is most unwholesome, and even dangerous.

Cellar and Kitchen Air. Houses in which fruit and vegetables are stored in the cellar become filled with very unpleasant odors from the decay of these. Others again, where the kitchen is not properly ventilated, get the smoke of frying and the smell of cooking all through them. But such sources of impurity, while injurious and always to be strictly avoided, are neither half so dangerous when they occur, nor one-tenth so common as the great chief cause of impure air--our breaths and the other gases from our bodies, with the germs they contain.

Drafts not Dangerous. Now comes the practical question, How are we to get rid of these breath-poisons? From the carelessness of builders, and the porous materials of which buildings are made, most houses are very far from air-tight, and a considerable amount of pure air will leak in around window-casings, door-frames, knot-holes, and other cracks, and a corresponding amount of foul air leak out. But this is not more than one-fifth enough to keep the air fresh when the rooms are even partially occupied, still less when they are crowded full of people. As each individual, breathing quietly, requires about four bushels of air (one and a half cubic yards) a minute, it is easy to see that, when there are ten or more people in a room, there ought to be a steady current of air pouring into that room; and when there are twenty or even forty people, as in an average schoolroom, the current of air (provided there is one) must move so fast to keep up the supply that the people in the room begin to notice it and call it "a draft." It would be difficult to ventilate a room for even four or five persons without producing, in parts of it, a noticeable draft of air. In fact, it is pretty safe to say that, if somebody doesn't feel a draft the room is not being properly ventilated. At one time this was considered a very serious drawback--drafts were supposed to be so dangerous. But now we know that a draft is only air in motion, and that air in motion is the only air that is sure to be pure. There is nothing to be afraid of in a draft which is not too strong, if you are clean outside and in, and reasonably vigorous. If the draft is too strong, move away from the window or the door. Colds are very seldom caught from the cold, pure air of a draft, but nearly always from the germs, or dirt, in the still, foul air of a tightly closed room. This fact has swept away the chief objection to the direct, or natural, method of ventilating through open windows.

Methods of Ventilation. Fortunately, as often happens, the simplest and most natural method of ventilation is the best one. Open the windows, and let the fresh air pour in. If there be any room which hasn't windows enough in it to ventilate it properly, it is unfit for human occupation, and is seldom properly lighted. Most elaborate and ingenious systems of ventilation have been devised and put into our larger houses, and public buildings like libraries, court-houses, capitols, and schools. Some of them drive the air into each room by means of a powerful steam, or electric, fan in the basement; others suck the used-up air out of the upper part of each room, thus creating an area of low pressure, to fill which the fresh air rushes in through air-tubes or around doors and windows. They have elaborate methods of warming, filtering, and washing the air they distribute. Some work fairly well, some don't; but they all have one common defect--that what they pump into the rooms is not fresh air, though it may conform to all the chemical tests for that article. "The proof of the pudding is in the eating," and fresh air is air that will make those who breathe it feel fresh, which the cooked and strained product of these artificial ventilating systems seldom does.

If they could be combined with the natural, window system of ventilation, they would be less objectionable; but the first demand of nearly all of them is that the windows must be kept shut for fear of breaking the circuit of their circulation. Any system of ventilation, or anything else, that insists on all windows being kept shut is radically wrong. It is only fair to say, however, that most of these systems of ventilation attempt the impossible, as well as the undesirable thing of keeping people shut up too long. No room can be, or ought to be, ventilated so that its occupants can stay in it all day long without discomfort. In ventilating, we ought to ventilate the people in the room, as well as the room itself. This can only be done successfully by turning the people out of doors, at least every two or three hours if grown-ups, and every hour or so if children. That is what school recesses are for, and they might well be longer and more frequent.

The first and chief thing necessary for the good ventilation of houses and schools is plenty of windows, which are also needed to give proper light for working purposes, and to let in the only ever-victorious enemy of germs and disease--sunlight.

Secondly, and not less important, the windows should fit properly, and be perfectly hung and balanced, so that the sash will come down at a finger's touch, stay exactly where it is put, and go up again like a feather, instead of having to be pried loose, wrested open, held in place with a stick, and shoved up, or down again, only with a struggle.

There should be, if possible, windows on two sides of every room, or, if not, a large transom opening into a hall which has plenty of windows in it. With this equipment and a good supply of heat, any room can be properly ventilated and kept so. But it will not ventilate itself. Ventilation, like the colors of the great painter Turner, must be "mixed with brains"; and those brains must be in the room itself, not down in the basement. In the schoolroom, each teacher and pupil should regard the ventilation of the room as the most important single factor in the success of their work. The teacher has a sensitive thermometer and guide in, first, her own feelings and, second, the looks and attention of her pupils. There should be vacant seats or chairs in every room so that those too near the window in winter can move out of the strong current of cold air.

Windows should reach well up toward the ceiling and be opened at the top, because the foul air given off from the lungs at the temperature of the body is warmer than the air of the room and consequently rises toward the ceiling. It is just as important in ventilation to let the foul air out as to let the fresh air in. In fact, one is impossible without the other. Air, though you can neither see it, nor grasp it, nor weigh it, is just as solid as granite when it comes to filling or emptying a room. Not a foot, not an inch of it can be forced into a room anywhere, until a corresponding foot or inch is let out of it somewhere.

Therefore, never open a window at the bottom until you have opened it at the top. If you do, the cold fresh air will pour in onto the floor, while the hot foul air will rise and bank up against the ceiling in a layer that gets thicker and thicker, and comes further and further down, until you may be actually sitting with your head and shoulders in a layer of warm foul air, and your body and feet in a pool of cool pure air. Then you will wonder why your head is so hot, and your feet so cold!

Currents and Circulation of Air. In fact, this tendency of hot air to rise, and of cold air to sink, or rush in and take its place, which is the mainspring of nature's outdoor system of ventilation, is one of our greatest difficulties when we wall in a tiny section of the universe and call it a room. The difficulty is, of course, greatest in winter time, when the only pure air there is--that out of doors--is usually cold. This is one of the few points at which our instincts seem to fail us. For when it comes to a choice between being warm or well ventilated, we are sadly prone to choose the former every time. Still we would much rather be warm and well ventilated than hot and stuffy, and this is what we should aim for.

The main problem is the cost of the necessary fuel, as it naturally takes more to heat a current of air which is kept moving through the room, no matter how slowly, than it does a room full of air which is boxed in, as it were, and kept from moving on after it has been warmed. The extra fuel, however, means the difference between comfort and stuffiness, between health and disease. Fortunately, the very same cold which makes a room harder to heat makes it easier to ventilate. When air is warmed, it expands and makes a "low pressure," which sucks the surrounding cooler air into it, as in the making of winds; so that the warmer the air inside the room, or the colder the air outside of it, which is practically the same thing, the more eagerly and swiftly will the outdoor air rush into it. So keen is this draft, so high this pressure, that some loosely-built houses and rooms, with only a few people in them, will in very cold weather be almost sufficiently ventilated through the natural cracks and leaks without opening a window or a door at all. And what is of great practical importance, an opening of an inch or two at the top of a window will admit as much fresh air on a cold day as an opening of a foot and a half in spring or summer, so swiftly does cold air pour in.

Bearing this in mind, and also that it is always best to ventilate through as many openings as possible, both to keep drafts of cold air from becoming too intense, and to give as many openings for the escape of the foul air as possible, there will be little difficulty in keeping any room which has proper window arrangements well ventilated in winter. An opening of an inch at the top of each of three windows is better than a three-inch opening at the top of one. But you must use your brains about it, watching the direction of the wind, and frequently changing the position of the window sashes to match the changes of heat in the room, or of cold outside.

No arrangement of windows, however perfect, is likely to remain satisfactory for more than an hour at a time, except in warm weather. This watchfulness and attention takes time, but it is time well spent. "Eternal vigilance" is the price of good ventilation, as well as of liberty; and you will get far more work done in the course of a morning by interrupting it occasionally to go and raise or lower a window, than you will by sitting still and slaving in a stuffy, ill-smelling room.

Plenty of Heat Needed. Any method of heating--open fireplace, stove, hot air, furnace, hot water, or steam--which will keep a room with the windows open comfortably warm in cold weather is satisfactory and healthful. The worst fault, from a sanitary point of view, that a heating system can have is that it does not give enough warmth, so that you are compelled to keep the windows shut. Too little heat is often as dangerous as too much; for you will insist on keeping warm, no matter what it may cost you in the future, and a cold room usually means hermetically sealed windows. Remember that coal is cheaper than colds, to say nothing of consumption and pneumonia.

Ventilating the Bedroom. The same principles that apply to ventilating a living-room or day-room apply to ventilating a bedroom. Here you can almost disregard drafts, except in the very coldest weather, and, by putting on plenty of covering, sleep three hundred days out of the year with your windows wide open and your room within ten degrees of the temperature outdoors. You need not be afraid of catching cold. On the contrary, by sleeping in a room like this you will escape three out of four colds that you usually catch. Sleeping with the windows wide open is the method we now use to cure consumption, and it is equally good to prevent it.

No bedroom window ought to be closed at the top, except when necessary to keep rain or snow from driving in. Close the windows for a short time before going to bed, and again before rising in the morning, to warm up the room to undress and dress in; or have a small inside dressing-room, with your bed out on a screened balcony or porch. But sleep at least three hundred nights of the year with the free air of heaven blowing across your face. You will soon feel that you cannot sleep without it. In winter, have a light-weight warm comforter and enough warm, but light, blankets on your bed, and leave the heat on in the room, if necessary--but open the windows.

COLDS, CONSUMPTION, AND PNEUMONIA

Disease Germs. In all foul air there are scores of different kinds of germs-- many of them comparatively harmless, like the yeasts, the moulds, the germs that sour milk, and the bacteria that cause dead plants and animals to decay. But among them there are a dozen or more kinds which have gained the power of living in, and attacking, the human body. In so doing, they usually produce disease, and hence are known as disease germs.

These germs--most of which are known, according to their shape, as bacilli ("rod-shaped" organisms), or as cocci (round, or "berry-shaped" organisms)-- are so tiny that a thousand of them would have to be rolled together in a ball to make a speck visible to the naked eye. But they have some little weight, after all, and seldom float around in the air, so to speak, of their own accord, but only where currents of air are kept stirred up and moving, without much opportunity to escape, and especially where there is a good deal of dust floating, to the tiny particles of which they seem to cling and be borne about like thistle-down. This is one reason why dusty air has always been regarded as so unwholesome, and why a very high death rate from consumption, and other diseases of the lungs, is found among those who work at trades and occupations in which a great deal of dust is constantly driven into the air, such as knife-grinders, stone-masons, and printers, and workers in cotton and woolen mills, shoddy mills, carpet factories, etc.

In cleaning a room and its furniture, it is always best to use a carpet sweeper, a vacuum cleaner, or a damp cloth, as much as possible, the broom as little as may be, and the feather duster never. The two latter stir up disease germs resting peacefully on the floor or furniture, and set them floating in the air, where you can suck them into your lungs.

There are three great groups of disease germs which may be found floating in the air wherever people are crowded together without proper ventilation-- for most of these disease germs cannot live long outside of the body, and hence come more or less directly from somebody else's lungs, throat, or nose. The most numerous, but fortunately the mildest group, of these are the germs of various sorts which give rise to colds, coughs, and sore throats. Then there are two other exceedingly deadly germs, which kill more people than any other disease known to humanity--the bacillus of consumption, and the coccus of pneumonia.

Our best protection against all these is, first, to have our rooms well ventilated, well lighted, and well sunned; for most of these germs die quickly when exposed to direct sunlight, and even to bright, clear daylight. The next most important thing is to avoid, so far as we can, coming in contact with people who have any of these diseases, whether mild or severe; and the third is to build up our vigor and resisting power by good food, bathing, and exercise in the open air, so that these germs cannot get a foothold in our throats and lungs.

Colds. Two-thirds of all colds are infectious, and due, not to cold pure air, but to foul, stuffy air, with the crop of germs that such air is almost certain to contain. They should be called "fouls," not "colds." They spread from one person to another; they run through families, schools, and shops. They are accompanied by fever, with headache, backache, and often chills; they "run their course" until the body has manufactured enough antitoxins to stop them, and then they get well of their own accord. This is why so many different remedies have a great reputation for curing colds.

If you "catch cold," stay in your own room or in the open air for a few days, if possible, and keep away from everybody else. You only waste your time trying to work in that condition, and will get better much more quickly by keeping quiet, and will at the same time avoid infecting anybody else. Get your doctor to tell you what mild antiseptic to use in your nose and throat; and then keep it in stock against future attacks. Often it is advisable to rest quietly in bed a few days, so as not to overtax the body in its weakened condition.

Keep away from foul, stuffy air as much as possible, especially in crowded rooms; bathe or splash in cool water every morning; sleep with your windows open; and take plenty of exercise in the open air; and you will catch few colds and have little difficulty in throwing off those that you do catch. Colds are comparatively trifling things in themselves; but, like all infections however mild, they may set up serious inflammations in some one of the deeper organs--lungs, kidneys, heart, or nervous system, and frequently make an opening for the entrance of the germs of tuberculosis or pneumonia. Don't neglect them; and if you find that you take cold easily, find out what is wrong with yourself, and reform your unhealthful habits.

HOW TO CONQUER CONSUMPTION

Different Forms of Tuberculosis. The terrible disease tuberculosis is the most serious and deadly enemy which the human body has to face. It kills every year, in the United States, over a hundred and fifty thousand men, women, and children--more lives than were lost in battle in the four years of our Civil War. It is caused by a tiny germ--the tubercle bacillus--so called because it forms little mustard-seed-like lumps, or masses, in the lungs, called tubercles, or "little tubers." For some reason it attacks most frequently and does its greatest damage in the lungs, where it is called consumption; but it may penetrate and attack any tissue or part of the body. Tuberculosis of the glands, or "kernels," of the neck and skin, is called scrofula; tuberculosis of the hip is hip-joint disease; and tuberculosis of the knee, white swelling. "Spinal disease" and "hunch-back" are, nine times out of ten, tuberculosis of the backbone. Tuberculosis of the bowels often causes fatal wasting away, with diarrhea, in babies and young children; and tuberculosis of the brain (called tubercular meningitis) causes fatal convulsions in infancy.

Tuberculosis of the Lungs--How to Keep it from Spreading. Tuberculosis of the lungs is the most dangerous of all forms, both because the lungs appear to have less power of resistance against the tubercle bacillus, and also because from the lung, the bacilli can readily be coughed up and blown into the air again, or spit onto the floor, to be breathed into the lungs of other people, and thus give them the disease. Two-thirds of all who die of tuberculosis die of the pulmonary, or lung, form of the disease, popularly called consumption.

The first thing then to be done to put a stop to this frightful waste of human life every year is to stop the circulation of the bacillus from one person to another. This can be done partially and gradually by seeing that every consumptive holds a handkerchief, or cloth, before his mouth whenever he coughs; that he uses a paper napkin, pasteboard box, flask, or other receptacle whenever he spits; and that these things in which the sputum is caught are promptly burned, boiled, or otherwise sterilized by heat. The only sure and certain way, however, of stopping its spread is by placing the consumptive where he is in no danger of infecting any one else. And as it fortunately so happens that such a place--that is to say, a properly regulated sanatorium, or camp--is the place which will give him his best chance of recovery, at least five times as good as if he were left in his own home, this is the plan which is almost certain to be adopted in the future. Its only real drawback is the expense.

But when you remember that consumption destroys a hundred and fifty thousand lives every year in this country alone, and that it is estimated that every human life is worth at least three thousand dollars to the community, you will see at once that consumption costs us in deaths alone, four hundred and fifty million dollars a year! And when you further remember that each person who dies has usually been sick from two to three years, and that two-thirds of such persons are workers, or heads of families, and that tens of thousands of other persons who do not die of it, have been disabled for months and damaged or crippled for life by it, you can readily see what an enormous sum we could well afford to pay in order to stamp it out entirely.

One of the most important safeguards against the disease is the law that prevents spitting in public places. Not only the germs of consumption, but those of pneumonia, colds, catarrhs, diphtheria, and other diseases, can be spread by spitting. The habit is not only dangerous, but disgusting, unnecessary, and vulgar, so that most cities and many states have now passed laws prohibiting spitting in public places, under penalty of fine and imprisonment.

The next best safeguard is plenty of fresh air and sunlight in every room of the house. These things are doubly helpful, both because they increase the vigor and resisting power of those who occupy the rooms and might catch the disease, and because direct sunlight, and even bright daylight, will rapidly kill the bacilli when it can get directly at them.

How great is the actual risk of infection in crowded, ill-ventilated houses is well shown by the reports of the tuberculosis dispensaries of New York and other large cities. Whenever a patient comes in with tuberculosis, they send a visiting nurse to his home, to show him how best to ventilate his rooms, and to bring in all the other members of the family to the dispensary for examination. No less than from one-fourth to one-half of the children in these families are found to be already infected with tuberculosis. The places where we look for our new cases of tuberculosis now are in the same rooms or houses with old ones. A careful consumptive is no source of danger; but alas, not more than one in three are of that character.

It has been estimated that any city or county could provide proper camps, or sanatoria, to accommodate all its consumptives and cure two-thirds of them in the process, support their families meanwhile, and stop the spread of the disease, at an expense not to exceed five dollars each per annum for five years, rapidly diminishing after that. If this were done, within thirty years consumption would probably become as rare as smallpox is now. Some day, when the community is ready to spend the money, this will be done, but in the mean time, we must attack the disease by slower and less certain methods.

Note the number of deaths from tuberculosis to one from smallpox; yet smallpox before the days of vaccination and quarantine, was the universal scourge. Similarly, by preventive measures, we are controlling the other diseases. Why not also tuberculosis? (Statistics for greater New York, 1908; total number of deaths from all causes, 73,072.

Why the Fear and Danger of Consumption have been Lessened. Terrible and deadly as consumption is, we no longer go about in dread of it, as people did twenty-five years ago, before we knew what caused it; for we know now that it is preventable and that two-thirds of the cases can be cured after they develop. The word consumption is no longer equivalent to a sentence of death. The deaths from tuberculosis each year have diminished almost one-half in the last forty years, in nearly every civilized country in the world; and this decrease is still going on.

The methods which have brought about this splendid progress, and which will continue it, if we have the intelligence and the determination to stick to them, are:--First, the great improvements in food supply, housing, ventilation, drainage, and conditions of life in general, due to the progress of modern civilization and science, combined with a marked increase in wages in the great working two-thirds of the community. Second, the discovery that consumption is caused by a bacillus, and by that alone, and is spread by the scattering of that bacillus into the air, or upon food, drink, or clothing, to be breathed in or eaten by other victims. Third, increase of medical skill and improved methods of recognizing the disease at a very early stage. A case of consumption discovered early means a case cured, eight times out of ten.

Its Cure and Prevention. Fortunately, the same methods which will cure the disease will also prevent it. The best preventatives are food, fresh air, and sunshine. Eat plenty of nourishing food three times a day, especially of milk, eggs, and meat. Sit or work in a gentle current of air, keep away from those who have the disease, sleep with your windows open, take plenty of exercise in the open air, and you need have little fear of consumption.

In the camps, or sanatoria, for the cure of consumption, these methods are simply carried a little further, to make up for previous neglect. The patients sit or lie out of doors all day long, usually in reclining chairs, in summer under the trees, and in winter on porches, with just enough roof to protect them from rain or snow. They sleep in tents, or in shacks, which are closed in only on three sides, leaving the front open to the south. They dress and undress in a warm room, or the curtains of the tent are dropped, or the shutters of the shack closed night and morning until the room is warmed up. In cold climates they dress day and night almost as if they were going on an arctic relief expedition, and spend twenty-four hours out of the twenty-four in the open air.

They eat three square meals a day, consisting of everything that is appetizing, nutritious, and wholesome, with plenty of butter, or other fats; and in addition, drink from one to three pints of new milk and swallow from six to twelve raw eggs a day. You would think they would burst on such a diet, but they don't; they simply gain from two to four pounds a week, lose their fever and their cough, get rid of their night sweats, and usually in from two to five weeks are able to be up and about the camp, taking light exercise. When they have reached their full, normal, or healthy weight for their height and age, their amount of food is reduced, but still kept at what would be considered full diet for a healthy man at hard work. If sick people can be made well by this open air treatment, those of us that are well ought not be afraid to have a window open all night.

Two-thirds of the treatment that would cure you of consumption will prevent your ever having it. While tuberculosis chiefly attacks the lungs, it is really a disease of the entire body, or system, and cannot attack you if you will keep yourself strong, vigorous, and clean in every sense of the word.

How to Recognize the Disease in its Early Stages. To recognize the disease early is, of course, work for the doctor; but he must be helped by the intelligence of the patient, or the patient's family, or he may not see the case until it is so far advanced as to have lost its best chance of cure. We can now recognize consumption before the lungs are seriously diseased. Among the most useful methods with children is the rubbing or scratching of a few drops of the toxin of the tubercle bacillus, tailed tuberculin, into the skin. If the children are healthy, this will leave no mark, or reddening, at all; but if they have tuberculosis, in two-thirds of the cases it will make a little reddening and swelling like a very mild vaccination. But in order to get any good from this, cases must be brought to a doctor, early, without waiting for a bad cough, or for night sweats.

Signs of Consumption. The signs that ought to make us suspicious of a possible beginning of tuberculosis are first, loss of weight without apparent cause; fever, or flushing of the cheeks, with or without headache, every afternoon or evening; and a tendency to become easily tired and exhausted without unusual exertion. Whenever these three signs are present, without some clear cause, such as a cold, or unusual overwork or strain, especially if they be accompanied by a rapid pulse and a tendency to get out of breath readily in running upstairs, they should make us suspect tuberculosis; and if they keep up, it is advisable to go at once and have the lungs thoroughly examined. Nine cases out of ten, seen at this stage, are curable--many of them in a few months.

Even if we should not have the disease, if we have these symptoms we need to have our health improved; and a course of life in the open air, good feeding, and rest, which would cure us if we had tuberculosis, will build us up and prevent us from developing it.

PNEUMONIA

Its Cause and Prevention. The other great disease of the lungs is pneumonia, formerly known as inflammation of the lungs. This is rapid and sudden, instead of slow and chronic like tuberculosis, but kills almost as many people; and unfortunately, unlike tuberculosis, is not decreasing. In fact in some of our large cities, it is rapidly increasing. Although we know it is due to a germ, we don't yet know exactly how that germ is conveyed from one victim to another. One thing, however, of great practical importance we do know, and that is that pneumonia is a disease of overcrowding and foul air, like tuberculosis; that it occurs most frequently at that time of the year--late winter and early spring--when people have been longest crowded together in houses and tenements; and that it falls most severely upon those who are weakened by overcrowding, under-feeding, or the excessive use of alcohol. How strikingly this is true may be seen from the fact that, while the death-rate of the disease among the rich and those in comfortable circumstances, who are well-fed and live in good houses, is only about five per cent,--that is, one in twenty,--among the poor, especially in the crowded districts of our large cities, the death-rate rises to twenty per cent, or one in five; while among the tramp and roustabout classes, who have used alcohol freely, and among chronic alcoholics, it reaches forty per cent. The same steps should be taken to prevent its spread as in tuberculosis--destroying the sputum, keeping the patient by himself, and thoroughly ventilating and airing all rooms. As the disease runs a very rapid course, usually lasting only from one to three weeks, this is a comparatively easy thing to do.

Though pneumonia is commonly believed to be due to exposure to cold or wet, like colds, it has very little to do with these. You will not catch pneumonia after breaking through the ice or getting lost in the snow, unless you already have the germs of the disease in your mouth and throat, and your constitution has already been run down by bad air, under-feeding, overwork, or dissipation. Arctic explorers, for instance, never catch pneumonia in the Frozen North.

CHAPTER XV

THE SKIN

OUR WONDERFUL COAT

What the Skin Is. The skin is the most wonderful and one of the most important structures in the body. We are prone to think lightly of it because it lies on the surface, and to speak of it as a mere coating, or covering--a sort of body husk; but it is very much more than this. Not only is it waterproof against wet, a fur overcoat against cold, and a water jacket against heat, all in one, but it is also a very important member of the "look-out department," being the principal organ of one of our senses, that of touch.

The eyes in the beginning were simply little colored patches of the skin, sunk into the head for the purpose of specializing on the light-rays. The smelling areas of the nose also were pieces of the skin, as were also the ears. Not only so, but--although it is a little hard for you to understand how this could have happened--the whole brain and nervous system is made up of folds of the skin tucked in from the surface of the back; so that we can say that the skin, with the organs that belong to it and have grown from it--the eyes, nose, ears, brain, and nerves--forms the most wonderful part of the body. Everything that we know of the world outside of us is told us by the skin and the look-out organs that have grown out of it. The skin is not only the surface part and coating of the body, far superior to any six different kinds of clothing which have yet been invented, but it is related to, and assists in, the work of nearly half the organs in the body. Not only all that we learn by touch and pressure, but everything that we know of heat and cold, of moisture and dryness, and most of pain, comes to us through our skin, through the little bulbs on the ends of the nerve twigs in it. It also helps the lungs to breathe, the kidneys to purify the blood, and the heart to control the flow of blood through the body.

A healthy skin is of very great importance; and part of this health we can secure directly, by washing and bathing, scrubbing and kneading and rubbing, because the skin lies right on the surface, where we can readily get at it. But, on the other hand, no amount of attention from the outside alone will keep it healthy. All the organs inside the body must be kept healthy if the skin is to be kept in good condition. Although the external washing and cleaning are very important, the greater part of the work of developing a healthy skin and a good complexion must be done from the inside.

The Two Layers which Make Up the Skin. Like our "internal skin," the mucous membrane, which lines our stomach and bowels, the skin is made up of two layers--a deeper, or basement, sheet, woven out of tough strands of fibrous stuff (derma); and a surface layer (epidermis) composed of cells lying side by side like the bricks in a pavement, or the tiles on a floor, and hence called "pavement" (epithelial) cells. These pavement cells are fastened on the basement membrane much as the kernels of corn grow on a cob; only, instead of there being but one layer, as on a cob of corn, there are a dozen or fifteen of them, one above the other, each one dovetailing into the row below it, as the corn kernels do into the surface of the cob. As they grow up toward the surface from the bottom, they become flatter and flatter, and drier, until the outer surface layer becomes thin, fine, dry, slightly greasy scales, like fish-scales, of about the thickness of the very finest and driest bran.

We are continually Shedding our Skin. One way in which the skin keeps itself so wonderfully clean and fresh is by continually shedding from its surface showers of these fine, dry, scaly cells, which drop, or are rubbed off, as they dry. This is the reason why no mark, not even a stain or dye, upon the skin, will stay there long; for no matter how deeply it may have soaked into the layers of the pavement-cells, every cell touched by it will ultimately grow up to the surface, dry up, and fall off, carrying the stain with it.

If you want to make a mark on the skin that will be permanent, you have to prick the colors into it so deeply that they will go through the basement layer and reach cells which will not grow toward the surface. This "pricking-in" operation is known as tattooing; and it is as foolish as it is painful, for blood-poisoning and other diseases may be carried into the system in the process.

Perhaps you will wonder why, if you are shedding these scales from all over your surface every day, you don't see them. This is simply because they are so exceedingly small, thin, and delicate, that you cannot see them unless you get a large number of them together; and when you are changing your clothing, bathing, etc., they are rubbed off and float away. If a part of the body has been shut in--as when a broken arm, for instance, is in a cast, which cannot be changed for several weeks--when finally you take off the bandage, you will find inside it spoonfuls--I had almost said handfuls--of fine scales, which have been shed from the skin and held in by the wrappings.

THE GLANDS IN THE SKIN

Sweat Glands. Like all the pavement (epithelial) surfaces of the body, inside and out, the skin has the power of making glands by dipping down little pouches or pockets into the layers below. In the skin, these little gland-pockets are of two kinds, the sweat glands and the hair glands.

The sweat glands are tiny tubes which go twisting down through the different pavement layers, through the basement layer, and right into the coat of fat, which lies just under the skin. The tube of the sweat gland soaks, or picks, out of the blood some of the waste-stuff--just as the kidney tube does in the kidney,--together with a good deal of water and a small amount of delicate oil, and pours them out on the surface of the body in the form of the "sweat," or perspiration.

As you will remember, when the muscles work hard and pour more waste into the blood, then the heart pumps larger amounts of blood out into the skin; and this causes it to redden. The sweat glands work harder to purify this extra blood, and they pour out the waste and oil and water on the surface. As soon as this water gets upon our hot skin, it begins to evaporate and cool us off, as well as to carry off some of the waste in the form of gas. The trace of oil in the perspiration helps to lubricate the skin and keep it soft; but when too much of it is poured out we have that greasy feeling, which we have all felt after perspiring freely.

From all this cooling and breathing and blood-purifying work going on upon the surface of our skin, you can easily see why it is so important that all our clothing should be loose and porous and that next the skin easily washed; else it will very soon become clogged up and greasy, and shut off the breathing and blood-purifying work of the skin and make it dirty and unhealthy. This continual mist of water, rising and bubbling up through our skin like springs out of a hillside, is another of nature's wonderful ways of cleansing the skin and of preventing any kind of dirt from permanently sticking to or lodging in it. Remember, you do not need to dig below the surface when you wash.

Hair Glands. The other kind of skin glands, the hair glands, are also pouches growing out from the deepest part of the stem of the hair, known as the root, or hair bulb.

From the root of the hairs, two or three little bundles of muscle run up toward the surface of the skin. When these contract, they pull the root of the hair up toward the surface, causing the hair to stand erect, or "bristle," as we say. This is what makes the hair on a dog's or a cat's back stand up when he is angry; but the commonest use of the movement is, when animals are cold, to make their coats stand out so as to hold more air and retain the body-heat better. We have lost most of our hairy coating, but whenever we get chilly, whether from cold or from fright, these little muscles of our hair bulbs contract and pull the hair glands of our skin up toward the surface, so that it looks all "pimply" or "goose-skinned."

Each hair pouch has sprouted out from its sides a pair of tiny pouches, which form oil glands to lubricate the hair and keep it sleek and flexible. It is hard to beat nature at her own game, and her method of oiling the hair is far superior to any hair oil that can be put on from the outside. Keep your hair well brushed and washed, and nature will oil it for you much better than any hair oil or scalp reviver ever invented.[19]

THE NAILS

How the Nails are Made. Another "trade," which our wonderful skin has literally "at its fingers' ends," is that of making nails. Indeed, every kind of scale, armor, fur, feather, and leather coating possessed by bird, beast, or fish was made by, and out of, the skin. Nail-making, however, is one of its simplest feats, as it is carried out merely by turning a little patch, or area, of itself into a horn-like substance. This, the skin of insects, of fishes, of crocodiles, etc., does all over the surface of their bodies; but in animals and birds only a number of little patches at the tips of the toes harden up in this way, to form the claws or nails; and in birds, the beak; and in some animals, the horns. So it is quite correct to call the substance of our nails "horn-like."

In some animals and birds, these little horny patches at the ends of the toes grow out into long, curved hooks, or broad, digging chisels and scoops; but on our own fingers, they simply make a little mould over the finger-tip. If, however, they are protected from being broken off, they will grow four or five inches long; in fact, they are carefully trained to do this by some of the upper classes in China, merely for the purpose of showing that they have never been obliged to degrade themselves, as they foolishly regard it, by working with their hands.

You can easily prove that the nails do grow constantly from the root or base, out toward the tip, by watching, some time when you have pounded one of your nails, how the black or discolored patch in it will grow steadily outward toward the tip, where it will be broken off and shed.

You cannot see the softest and youngest row, or layer, of the nail cells at the base, because a fold of skin, the nail fold, has been doubled, or folded, over them to protect them while they are young and soft. It is not best to push this fold of skin back too much, as, by so doing, you may uncover the young nail cells while they are soft and tender, and expose them to injury. The reason why there is a little whitish crescent at the base of the nail is that the cells of the nail do not grow hard and horn-like and transparent until they have grown out a quarter of an inch or so from under the fold, but at first look whitish, or opaque, like the rest of the skin.

Health Shown by the Color of the Nails. Your nails and your lips are not really any redder, or pinker, than the rest of your skin; but the cells forming them are clear and transparent and allow the red blood to show through. This is why we often look at the nails and lips to see what the color of the blood is like, and how well or badly it is circulating. If the blood is anemic, or thin, then both lips and nails are pale and dull. If the blood is healthy and the circulation good, then the nails are pink, and the lips clear red. If, on the other hand, the circulation is bad, as in some forms of lung disease and heart disease, so that the blood is loaded with carbonic acid until it is blue and dark, then the lips may become purplish or dark blue, and the finger nails nearly the same color.

THE BLOOD-MESH OF THE SKIN

The Blood Vessels under the Skin. Not merely the nails and the lips, but the whole surface of the skin is underlaid with a thick mat, or network, of blood vessels. These vessels are all quite small, so that a cut has to go down completely through the skin, and generally well down into the muscles, before it will reach any blood vessel which will bleed at a dangerous rate. But there are so many of them, and they cover such a wide surface throughout the body, that they are actually capable of holding, at one time, nearly one-tenth of all the blood in the body.

This "water-jacket" coat of tiny blood vessels all over our body has some very important uses: It allows the heart to pump large amounts of blood out to the surface to be purified by the sweat glands, and to breathe out a little of its carbon dioxid and other gas-poisons.

The Skin as a Heat Regulator. Heat, as well as waste, is given off by the blood when it is poured out to the surface; so another most important use of the skin is as a heat regulator. As we have already seen, every movement which we make with our muscles, whether of arms and limbs, heart, or food tube, causes heat to be given off. We very well know, when we work hard at anything, we are likely to "get warmed up." Although a certain amount of this heat is necessary to our bodily health, too much of it is very dangerous.

Just as it is best for the temperature, or heat, of a room to be at about a certain level, somewhere from 60?to 70?F., so it is best for the interior of our bodies to be kept at about a certain heat. This, as we can show by putting a little glass thermometer under the tongue, or in the armpit, and holding it there for a few minutes, is a little over 98?F. (98.4?to be exact); and this we call "body heat," or "blood heat," or "normal temperature." Our body cells are, in one way, a very delicate and sensitive sort of hot-house plants, though tough enough in other respects. Whenever our body heat goes down more than five or six degrees, or up more than two or three degrees, then trouble at once begins. If our temperature goes down, as from cold or starvation, we begin to be drowsy and weak, and finally die. If, on the other hand, our temperature climbs up two, three, or four degrees, then we begin to be dizzy and suffer from headache and say we have "a fever."

A fever, or rise of temperature, that can be noted with a thermometer, is usually due to disease germs of some sort in the body; and most of the discomfort that we suffer is really due more to the poisons (toxins) of the germs than to the mere increase of heat, though this alone will finally work serious damage. However, as we well know from repeated experience, we need only to run or work hard in the sun for a comparatively short time to make ourselves quite hot enough to be very uncomfortable; and if we had no way to relieve ourselves by getting rid of some of this heat, we should either have to stop work at once, or become seriously ill. This relief, however, is just what nature has provided for in this thick coat of blood vessels in our skin; it enables us to throw great quantities of blood out to the surface where it can get rid of, or, as the scientists say, "radiate," its heat. This cooling process is hastened by the evaporation of the perspiration poured out at the same time, as we have seen.

One of the chief things in training for athletics is teaching our skin and heart together to get rid of the heat made by our muscles, as fast, or nearly as fast, as we make it, thus enabling us to keep on running, or working, without discomfort. As soon as we stop running, or working, the heart begins to slow down, the blood vessels in the skin contract and diminish in size, the flush fades, and we begin to cool off. We are not making either as much heat or as much waste as we were, and hence do not need to get rid of so much through our skins.

When we feel cold, just the opposite kinds of change occur in the skin. The blood vessels in the skin contract so as to keep as much of our warm blood as possible in the deeper parts of our body, and prevent its losing heat. As blood showing through the pavement-layer of the skin is what gives us our color, or complexion, our skin becomes pale and pasty-looking; and if all the blood is driven in from the surface, our lips and finger nails will become blue with cold. Here again, by changes in the skin, nature is simply trying to protect herself from the loss of too much heat.

If we exercise briskly, or eat a good warm meal, and thus make more heat inside of our body, then there is no longer any need to save its surface loss in this way; and the blood vessels in our skin fill up, the heart pumps harder, and the warm, rich color comes back to our faces and lips and finger nails.

So perfectly and wonderfully does this skin mesh of ours work, by increasing or preventing the loss of heat, that it is almost impossible to put a healthy man under conditions that will raise or lower his temperature more than about a degree, that is to say, about one per cent above, or below, its healthful level. Men studying this power of the skin have shut themselves into chambers, or little rooms, built like ovens, with a fire in the wall or under the floor, and found that if they had plenty of water to drink and perspired freely, they could stand a temperature of over 150?F. without great discomfort and without raising the temperature of their own bodies more than about one degree. If, however, the air in the chamber was moistened with the vapor of water, or steam, so that the perspiration could no longer evaporate freely from the surface of their bodies, then they could not stand a temperature much above 108?or 110?without discomfort.

Other men, who were trained athletes, have been put to work in a closed chamber, at very vigorous muscular exercise, so as to make them perspire freely. But while a thermometer placed in that chamber showed that the men were giving off enormous amounts of heat to the air around them, another thermometer placed under their tongues showed that they were raising the temperature of their own bodies only about half a degree. One man, however, happened to try this test one morning when he was not feeling very well, and didn't perspire properly, and the thermometer under his tongue went up nearly four degrees.

THE NERVES IN THE SKIN

How We Tell Things from Touch, and Feel Heat and Cold and Pain. Last of all, the skin is the principal organ of the sense of touch, and also of the "temperature sense"--the sense of heat and cold--and of the sense that feels pain. All these feelings are attended to by little bulbs lying in the deeper part of the skin and forming the tips of tiny nerve twigs,[20] which run inward to join larger nerve branches and finally reach the spinal cord. There are millions of these little bulbs scattered all over the surface of the skin, but they are very much thicker and more numerous in some parts than in others; and that is why, as you have often noticed, certain parts of the skin are more sensitive than others. They are thickest, for instance, on the tips of our fingers and on our lips, and fewest over the back of the neck and shoulders, and across the lower part of the hips.[21]

For a long time, it was supposed that all these little nerve-bulbs in the skin did the same kind of work, because they looked, under the microscope, exactly alike; but it was found that they divide the work up among them, so that some of them give their entire attention to heat, and others to cold, others to touch, and others again to pain. So carefully has the work been mapped out among them that they report to different centres in the brain and spinal cord, so that we now understand why, in diseases which happen to attack one or other of these centres, we may lose our sense of heat and cold, as in that terrible disease, leprosy; or our sense of touch, as in paralysis; or we may even, in some very rare cases, lose our sense of pain, and yet have all our other senses perfect.

FOOTNOTES:

[19] Hairs are of value chiefly as protection against cold and wet, although we have got rid of them and substituted clothing for this purpose, except on the top of our heads; but their roots also are very richly supplied with nerves so that they form almost a sort of feelers, or organs of sense. Many animals that move about much in the dark, like cats and bats, for instance, have their lips or faces studded with long, delicate, stiff hairs called whiskers, which act in this way and prevent their bumping into objects in the dark. And it is probable that the bristling of the hair on a dog's back, when he is angry or frightened, is in part for this purpose--to enable him to slip aside and dodge a blow, even after it has touched the ends of the hairs. This great sensitiveness of the hair roots is what makes it hurt so when any one pulls your hair.

[20] See the diagram of the skin on page 171.

[21] You can easily test this by a very simple experiment. Take a pair of dividers; or, if you haven't these, a couple of long pins or needles will do. Set them with their points a quarter of an inch apart. Then touch these points, first closing your eyes, so that you will not be able to see them, to the tip of one of your fingers, and you will readily feel that two points touch the skin. Turn your hand over and touch the back of it with the two points, and they will feel like one point. Carry the test further, over other parts of the body, and you will find that they are much less sensitive; thus you will find that at the back of the neck, or over the shoulder-blades, you will have to put the points nearly an inch apart before you can tell that there are two of them. This simply means that you have to touch two separate touch bulbs before you can get the idea of "two-ness." As these bulbs are an inch or more apart in the skin of the back, you have to spread the points of the dividers that

distance. You can also prove that the touching of two nerve-buds gives the idea of "two-ness" by crossing two of your fingers and placing a pea, or small round piece of chalk, between their crossed tips. If you close your eyes and roll the pea on the table, or desk, you will think you have two peas between your fingers.

CHAPTER XVI

HOW TO KEEP THE SKIN HEALTHY

CLOTHING

Clothes should be Loose and Comfortable. Man is the only animal that has no natural suit of clothing. Birds have feathers, and animals have fur, or hair, which they shed in summer and thicken up in winter without even thinking about it, so that they do not have to bother with either overcoats or flannels. The wise men say that man originally had a full suit of hair like other animals, and that he gradually got rid of it, as he became human. Whether this be true or not, the fact remains that he has none now; and consequently he must invent and manufacture something to take its place.

Originally, in the time of our savage ancestors, clothing was worn chiefly as protection from cold at night, so that all the earlier forms of clothing were of a more or less blanket-or cloak-like form, and wrapped, or swathed, the whole body without fitting closely to the limbs. It is interesting to remember this fact, because even our most highly civilized forms of clothing still show this same tendency. The skirt, for instance, is simply a survival of the lower end of the blanket, which has never been cut down to fit the limbs.

The principles upon which garments should be built are two: First, they should fit closely enough to the body and limbs to protect them from either injury or cold, even while free activity of every sort is allowed--you could not wrestle in a blanket or run very far in a sack. Second, they should be thick enough to protect us from cold, and yet at the same time porous enough not to interfere with the natural breathing and ventilating of the skin. A garment should be as loose as possible without interfering with our movements, and as free and as light as can be worn with reasonable warmth and protection. The less clothing you can wear and be comfortable, the better.

We should particularly avoid binding or cramping the chest and the hips and waist. If clothing is too tight about the chest, it interferes both with free movement of the arms and, what is even more important, with the breathing movements of the chest. If too tight about the waist and hips, it badly cripples the lower limbs and interferes with the proper movements of the diaphragm in breathing, and with the passage of the food and the blood through the bowels.

Your instincts are perfectly right that make you dislike to be squeezed or pinched or cramped in any way, or at any point, by your clothing; and if you will only follow these instincts all through your lives, you will be far healthier and happier.

The Texture of Clothing. Just as for ages we have experimented with different kinds of food, so we have with different kinds of material for clothing. We have used the skins of animals; mats woven out of leaves and grasses; the feathers of birds; the skins of fishes; cloths made of wool and of cotton; and even the cocoon spun by certain caterpillars, which we call silk. But of all these materials, practically only two have stood the test of the ages and proved themselves the most suitable and best all-round clothing materials--wool and cotton.

Woolen cloth, woven from the fleece of sheep or goats or camels or llamas or alpacas, has three great advantages, which make it the outside clothing of the human species. First, it is sufficiently tough and lasting to withstand rips and tugs and ordinary wear and tear; second, it is warm--that is, it retains well the body heat; and third, it is porous, so that it will allow gases and perspiration from the surface of the body to pass through it in one direction, and air for the skin to breathe, in the other.

No clothing, of course,--not even fur,--has any warmth in itself; it simply has the power of retaining, or keeping in, the warmth of the body that it covers. The best and most effective way of retaining the body warmth is to surround the body with a layer of dead, or still, air, which is the best non-conductor of heat known. Hence, porous garments, like loosely-woven flannels, blankets, and other woolen cloths, are warm because they contain or hold large amounts of air in their spongy mesh.

The reason why furs are so warm is that their soft, furry under-hairs, or "pelt" as the furriers call it, entangle and hold an enormous amount of air. The fur of ordinary sealskin, for instance, is about half an inch deep; and ninety per cent of this half-inch is air. If you wet it, its fur "slicks down" to almost nothing, although the most drenching wetting will not wash all the air out of it, but still leaves a dry layer next to the skin. The fur of mink skin, coon skin, or wolf skin, is an inch thick; and nearly eighty per cent of this thickness is air.

The great advantage for clothing purposes of wool over fur is that the wool is porous through and through, while the fur is borne upon, and backed by, a layer of leather--the skin of the animal upon which it grew--which layer, after tanning and curing, becomes almost absolutely air-tight.

As a matter of fact, furs are worn mostly for display and are most unwholesome and undesirable garments. The only real excuse for their use, save for ornament in small pieces or narrow strips, is on long, cold rides in the winter, and among lumbermen, frontiersmen, and explorers. They hold in every particle of perspiration and poisonous gas thrown off by the skin, and if worn constantly, make it pale, weak, and flabby; and the moment we take them off, we take cold.

For outer garments and general wear, nothing yet has been discovered equal to wool, particularly at the cooler times of the year. But for under wear, in the hotter seasons and climates, wool has certain disadvantages. It is likely to be rough and tickling to most skins, which makes it uncomfortable, especially in warm weather. It is also difficult and troublesome to wash woolens without shrinking them; and, as soon as they do shrink, not only do they become uncomfortably tight, but the natural pores in them which make them so valuable close up, and they become almost air-tight. Finally, when loaded with perspiration, woolens easily become offensive, so that they must be frequently changed and washed; and as they are also high in price, it is easily seen that there are practical drawbacks to their use.

Cotton is much softer and pleasanter to the skin than wool, is cooler in hot weather, is much cheaper, and is very easily washed without losing either its shape or its porousness. It can be so woven as to be almost as porous as wool, and to retain that porousness even when saturated with perspiration. It does not soak up and retain the oils and odors of perspiration in the way that wool does; and on the whole, for under wear, and for general wear at the warm seasons of the year, it is not only more comfortable, but far more healthful, than wool. Persons of fair health and reasonably vigorous outdoor habits, whose skins are well bathed and ventilated, can wear properly woven cotton or linen undergarments the whole year round with perfect safety.

Linen and silk both make admirable and healthful under wear, if woven with a properly porous mesh. Linen has the advantage of remaining more porous than cotton, when moist with perspiration. But for healthy people they have no advantages over cotton that are not offset by their higher prices.

BATHS AND BATHING

Bathing as a Means of Cleanliness. It has been said that one of the reasons why man lost his hairy coat was that he might be able to wash himself better and keep cleaner. However this may be, he has to wash a great deal oftener than other animals, most of whom get along very well with currying, licking, and other forms of dry washes, and an occasional swim in a river or lake.

You can readily see how necessary for us washing is, when you remember the quarts of watery perspiration, which are poured out upon our skins every day, and the oily and other waste matters, some of them poisons, which the perspiration leaves upon our skins. Especially is some means of washing necessary when the free evaporation of perspiration and the free breathing of the skin has been interfered with by clothing which is water-tight or too thick.

Bathing as a Tonic. But bathing is of much greater value than simply as a means of cleansing. Splashing the body with water is the most valuable means that we have of toning up and hardening the skin, and protecting us against the effects of cold. The huge and wonderfully elaborate network of blood vessels that lies in and just under our skins all over our bodies is, from the point of view of circulation, second only in importance to our hearts, and from the point of view of taking cold, and of resisting the attack of disease, one of the most important structures in our entire body. If, by means of daily baths, you keep this mesh of blood vessels in your skin toned up, vigorous, and elastic, and full of red blood, it will do more to keep you in perfect health and vigor than almost any other one thing, except an abundance of food, and plenty of fresh air and exercise. A healthy skin is the best undergarment ever invented.

Right and Wrong Bathing. The best form of bath is either the tub or the shower bath; and the cooler the water, provided that you warm up to it quickly and pleasantly, the greater the tonic effect, the more exhilaration and pleasure you will get out of it, and the more it will harden your skin against cold. But it should never under any circumstances be any cooler than you can readily and pleasantly react, or warm up to, during the bath and afterward. The habit of plunging into a great tub of ice-cold water all winter long, except for people of vigorous constitutions and active habits, may often do quite as much harm as good. Have your bath water just cool enough to give you a slight, pleasant shock, as you plunge into it, or turn it on, so that you will enjoy the glow and sense of exhilaration that follows; and you will get all the good there is out of the cold bath, and none of the harm. By beginning with moderately cool water you will find that you come to enjoy it cooler and cooler. If a bath-room is not at hand, a large wash-bowl of cool, or cold, water into which you can dip your hands and splash well over the upper half of your body every morning, and once or twice a week all over your body, will keep your skin clean and vigorous. If you cannot warm up properly after a cool bath, there is something wrong about your habits of life; and you had better change them, and keep changing them, until you find you can enjoy it. For some delicate children, a quick plunge into, or splash with, very hot water in the morning will give somewhat the same tonic effect as stronger ones can get from cold water.

[Illustration: AS A TONIC, SWIMMING IS THE BEST FORM OF BATHING]

Warm baths are best taken at night, just before going to bed, though the danger of catching cold after them on account of their "opening up the pores of the skin," has been very greatly exaggerated. They have, however, a relaxing effect upon the skin, and take out an undue amount of the natural oil which nature provides for its oiling and softening, so that, except for special reasons, it is best not to take them oftener than once, or twice, a week.

Soaps and Scrubbing Brushes. As part of the perspiration deposited upon our skins is in the form of a delicate oil, and as this oil may become mixed with dirt, or dust, and form a mixture not readily soluble in water, it is at times advisable to add to the water something that will dissolve oil. The commonest thing used for this purpose is soap, which is a combination of an alkali--most commonly soda, though occasionally potash (lye) is used in the soft soaps--with a fat or an oil. The combination of the two, which we call soap, has been invented for two reasons; one, that it makes a convenient, solid form in which the alkali, needed to dissolve the body oil, can be used in such strength as not to burn or injure the skin; the other, that the fat in the soap will, to some extent, take the place of the natural oil, or fat, which it washes off.

Necessary as soap is, it should be used very moderately. You should never lather and scrub your skin as if it were a kitchen floor, for the reason that, with the dirt, the alkali also washes and dissolves out a considerable amount of the natural oil of the skin, and leaves it harsh and dry. On this account, it is best not to use soap upon the covered portions of the body, and in the full bath, oftener than once or twice a week; and upon the face, oftener than once or twice a day. But the hands may be washed with soap more frequently.

It is also best to avoid the too frequent use of hot water, even upon the hands and face, for the same reason; it takes out too much of the natural oil of the skin, along with the dirt. Unless the dirt be of some infectious, or offensive, character, it is often best to content yourself with washing off just the "big dirt," and wait for the bubbling up of the perspiration through your skin to bring the deeper dirt up to the surface, and wash that off later, in the course of two or three hours.

Soaps to be Avoided. Soaps that lather too quickly and easily should always be avoided, for this shows that they contain an excessive amount of soda or other alkali. It is also best to avoid, or at least be very wary of, any soaps which are dark-colored or heavily perfumed, as these disguises may indicate the presence of decaying, offensive fats, and even of grease extracted from garbage. This is what strong perfumes in soaps are chiefly used for. Beware of all such, and especially of tar soaps, for the black color and the strong odor of tar can cover up any amount of bad quality.

Medicated soaps (soaps containing medicines) are also best let alone. They are only fit to be used on the advice of a doctor. Most of them are out and out humbugs, and make up for their richness in drugs by their poorness in good, pure fat and alkali. Moreover, what may suit one particular diseased condition of the skin is quite as likely to be injurious as helpful to another. Any drug which has the power of curing disease is almost certain to be irritating to a healthy skin; and nothing can be put into a soap beyond pure, sweet fat, or oil, and good soda, which will make it any better, or more wholesome, for a healthy skin. If your skin be red, or itchy, or scaly, or out of condition in any way, go to a doctor and get the appropriate treatment for that particular disease, instead of smearing on the surface of your body some drug of which you know nothing, in the hope of its being the proper thing for the little patch of diseased skin.

Avoid Using Skin Brushes. Scrubbing brushes and skin brushes of all sorts should be used even more sparingly than soap or hot water, for the same reason. Nature did not coat us over with either boards or rubber, but with delicate, velvety, sensitive, living skin worth ten times as much as any sort of leather, bark, rubber, or cloth, for resisting cold, heat, and injuries. It is most important for the health of the skin that we keep that velvety coating unscratched and unbroken. The use of brushes and bristles of all sorts, therefore, should be chiefly restricted to the hair and the finger nails, as for every ounce of dirt that they take out of the skin, they do a pound of damage to it. They scrub off the delicate epidermis, as well as the natural oil in it, and leave it dry and irritated and ready to crack open. Then more dirt gets into the cracks just formed, and more scrubbing with bristles and hot water and soap is indulged in to get it out. This opens the cracks still further, and the next layer of dirt is worked in still deeper. Wash frequently with cold or cool water, occasionally with hot water, and sparingly with soap; and limit the use of brushes to the nails and the hair.

CARE OF THE NAILS

Importance of Clean Nails. On account of their constant use, your hands are brought in contact with dusty or dirty substances in your work and in your play; and it is very easy for some of this dirt, and such germs as it may contain, to lodge in the little chink under the free edge of the nail, between it and the rounded end of the finger. It is of great importance that this nail chink should be kept clean, not only because it looks both ugly and untidy to have the ends of your fingers "in mourning," with black bands across them, but also because the germs lodged under your nails may get onto your food the next time that you eat, and set up irritation and fermentation in your stomach. They may also cause other trouble; for instance, if your collar chafes the back of your neck, and to relieve the itching you rub it a little too hard with your finger, your nail may scratch the skin; and if it be blackened with infectious dirt, this may get into the little scratch and give rise to a boil, or a festering sore.

How to Clean the Nails. This cleaning of the nails, however, must be done carefully and gently; for, if too harsh methods are used, the delicate skin on the under surface of the nail will be torn, the nail will be roughened or split, the dirt will work in just that much deeper next time, and the germs in it may set up inflammations under the nail. For this reason it is best not to use a sharp-pointed knife in cleaning the nails, but a blunt-pointed nail cleaner, such as can be bought for a few cents at any drug store, or such as many pocket-knives are now provided with. It is also best to trim the nails with a file or with scissors, instead of a knife, as the latter may split or tear the nail, or cut down to the quick. Before any of these are used, the nails should be thoroughly softened in warm water, and scrubbed with a moderately stiff nailbrush, such as should be kept on every washstand.

It is also best not to push back the fold of skin at the base of the nails, with instruments of any sort; or indeed, with anything harder than the ball of the thumb or finger. This fold protects the delicate growing part, or root, of the nail; and if it is shoved back too vigorously, the root may become exposed, or even inflamed and infected, and cause one of those extremely irritating little sores known as a "hangnail."

DISEASES AND DISTURBANCES OF THE SKIN

Their Chief Causes. Skin troubles are of two main kinds according to their cause: internal, due to the irritation of waste-poisons, or toxins, in the blood; and external, from direct injury or irritation of the skin from without.

The latter are often due to the wearing of too tight or too heavy clothing, or the failure properly to wash, cleanse, and ventilate the skin. Some of the lesser disturbances come from the chafing of collars, wristlets, and belts, and are, of course, relieved by loosening the clothing or substituting soft, comfortable cotton for rasping flannels. Others come from the use of too strong soaps, or the too frequent use of hot water, or too vigorous scrubbing of the skin, and these can be relieved by the avoidance of their cause.

Sunburn and Freckles and how to Cure Them. Upon the hands and face, sunburn and freckles may occur from exposure to the weather. They are not caused necessarily by exposure to direct sunlight; as the bright light and the cold air out of doors, also, will produce this irritating effect upon the skin.

The best way to cure sunburn is to bathe in cool water, take a night's rest, then go out the next day, and the day after, and take another dose of exposure, keeping this up until your face is hardened to stand a reasonable amount of sun. If you are in proper condition, neither your face nor your hands will sunburn uncomfortably. If they do, except under extreme exposure, it is a sign that you have not been living out of doors enough.

The various face-washes and creams and dusting powders which are used for the relief of sunburn, while they may, if mild enough, make the face feel somewhat more comfortable for a little time, owe most of their virtues to the fact that they are generally used at bedtime and then get the credit for the cure which nature works while you are asleep. If you should buy them, and keep them on your dressing-table unopened, where you could see them before you went to bed, you would in nine cases out of ten be just as much better in the morning as if you had used them.

The only harm done by freckles is to your vanity. They and sunburn both, in fact, are protective actions on nature's part, filling the skin with coloring matter, or pigment, so as to protect it, and the tissues below, from the irritating effects of the strong rays of light.

A like deposit of pigment, in greater amounts, in the skins of races who live in or near the tropics, gives rise to the characteristic coloring of the black, brown, and yellow races. The pigment, or coloring matter, is of exactly the same kind in all, from the negro to the white. The brown race having a little less of it than the negro, the yellow race a little less yet, and the white least of all, though there is some of it in even the whitest of skins.

Real Skin Diseases. Most of the serious and lasting diseases of the skin are caused by the attack of germs. Perfect cleanliness and ventilation are the best protection against them all; but if you should be unfortunate enough to catch one of these diseases, your doctor will be able to give you the mild germicide or antiseptic that will kill the particular germ that may have lodged upon your skin.

The commonest form of inflammation of the skin is called eczema, and eight-tenths of all eczemas are due to some mild germ, and can be cured by the appropriate poison for it.

Other diseases, particularly of the scalp, such as ringworm and dandruff, are due to other forms of vegetable germs, and may be cured by their proper poisons; while others, such as the so-called "prairie itch" (scabies), and lice in the hair, are due to the presence of tiny animal parasites.

The Hookworm. Another disease which enters through the skin is the now famous hookworm, or blood-sucking parasite, which has been found to be so common in tropical regions and in our Southern States. This parasite has the curious habit of attaching itself by hooks surrounding its mouth (which gave it its name), to the lining of the human intestine, particularly its upper third. There it swings, and lives by sucking the blood of its victim. When the worm has once attached itself in the intestine, it may live for from five to fifteen years. All this time it is constantly laying eggs; and these eggs, which are so tiny that they have to be put under a microscope to be seen, pass out in the feces; and if they are not deposited in a proper water closet, or deep vault, but scattered about upon the surface of the soil, the eggs quickly hatch into tiny, little wriggling worms called larv? which are still scarcely large enough to be seen with the naked eye.

These larv?live in the soil; and, when it is wet and muddy, they get up between the toes of boys and girls who are going barefoot, burrow their way in through the skin, and produce a severe itching inflammation of the skin of the feet, known as "ground-itch," "toe-itch" or "dew-itch." When they have worked their way through the skin, they bore on into a blood vessel, are carried to the heart, pumped by the heart into the lungs, and there again work their way out of the blood vessels into the bronchial, or air tubes, crawl up these through the windpipe and voice organ into the throat, are swallowed into the stomach, and from there pass on into the upper intestine to attach themselves for their blood-sucking life. If they are sufficiently numerous, their victim becomes thin, weak, and bloodless, with pale, puffy skin, and shortness of breath; he is easily tired on the least exertion, and ready to fall a victim to any disease, like tuberculosis, pneumonia, or typhoid, that may happen to attack him.

Their spread can be absolutely prevented either by the strict use of toilets or deep vaults, thus preventing the deposit of feces anywhere upon the surface of the ground; or by the constant wearing of shoes or sandals, thus preventing the larv?from attacking the feet and working their way through the skin and body into the intestine.

Fortunately, the disease is as curable as it is common, and two doses of a proper germicide, with a day in bed, and a laxative, will promptly cure it except in the worst cases.

The Rashes of Measles, Scarlet Fever, etc. Many of the infectious fevers, such as measles, scarlet fever, chicken-pox, and smallpox, are attended by rashes, or eruptions, upon the surface of the skin, due to a special gathering or accumulation of the particular germs causing each disease, just under the skin. When the skin sheds, or flakes off, after the illness, the germs are shed in the scales and float, or are carried about, and thus spread the disease to others.

These rashes or eruptions are not dangerous in themselves, though often very uncomfortable, but help us to recognize the disease; they probably show us the sort of thing that is going on in the deeper parts of the body. If you imagine that your throat and bronchial tubes and lungs are peppered as full of the disease spots as your skin is, in measles and in scarlet fever, you will readily understand why your throat is so sore and why you have so much tickling and coughing.

The Health of the Scalp and Hair. The scalp, being covered by hair, does not perspire so freely as the rest of the skin of the body; but a considerable amount of oily waste matter is poured out on it, and the surface of its skin scales off in exactly the same way as does the rest of the body. If this accumulation of tiny scales and grease is not properly brushed out, it forms an excellent seed-bed for some of the milder kinds of germs that attack the skin; and a scurfy, itchy condition of the scalp is set up, known as dandruff.

The best way to keep the scalp clean of these accumulations of greasy scales is by vigorous and regular brushing with a moderately stiff, but flexible, bristle brush. Wire brushes should not be used, as the wires scratch and irritate the delicate scalp and do more harm than good. If you watch a groom brushing and currying the coat of a thoroughbred horse, you will get a fair idea of hew you ought to treat your own scalp at least twice a day, night and morning.

If this currying of the hair be thoroughly done, and the head washed with soap and hot water about once a week for short hair and twice a month for long hair, most of the dangers of dandruff and of other infections of the scalp will be avoided. One thing to be remembered is, don't brush too hard or too deep. There is an old saying and a good one, "You can't brush the scalp too little, or the hair too much."

Wetting the hair for the purpose of "slicking" it or combing it, is about as bad a thing as could be done; for the moisture sets up a sort of rancid fermentation in the natural oil of the scalp, giving the well-known sour smell to hair that is combed instead of brushed, and furnishing a splendid soil for germs and bugs of all sorts to breed in. There is no objection to boys' and men's wetting their hair in cold water as often as they wish, provided that they rub it thoroughly dry afterward and give it a brisk currying with the brush.

Hair oils and greases of all sorts are sanitary nuisances, and mere half-civilized and lazy substitutes for proper brushing and washing. There is no drug known to medicine which will cause hair to grow, or make it thicker or curlier. All "hair tonics" claiming to do this are frauds.

Corns, Calluses, and Warts. Our skin not only made our hair, teeth, and nails, but still retains in every part a trace of its nail-making powers, so that under pressure or irritation, it can thicken up into a heavy leather-like substance which we call callus. This is naturally and healthfully present in the soles of the feet and the palms of the hands. Savage, or barbarous, races who wear no shoes get the skin of their soles thickened into a regular human leather, almost half an inch thick, and as tough as rawhide. A somewhat similar condition develops in the palms of the hands of those who work hard with spades, axes, or other tools.

Any good process carried to excess becomes bad, and this is true of this power of callus formation in the skin; for parts of it which are under constant pressure, like the surface of the toes inside the shoe, and particularly of the outside toes, the little and the big toe, develop under that pressure patches of thickened, horny skin, which we call corns. These patches start to grow into cone-shaped projections or buttons; but being prevented from growing outward by the pressure of the shoe, they turn upon themselves and burrow into the skin itself, and we get the well-known ingrowing corn.

If there is anything in the human body which we ought to be thoroughly ashamed of, it is corns; for they are caused by our own vanity, and nothing else, in cramping our feet into shoes one or two sizes too small for them. There are a number of things that can be done to relieve the discomfort of the corn, but the only sure way is to remove its cause, namely, the tight shoe.

Under other kinds of irritation, the skin has the power of growing curious little button-like buds, or projections, which we call warts. These are commonest in childhood, and generally disappear at about twelve or fifteen years of age, when we no longer delight in dirt, and glory in mud pies.

They can be produced upon the hands of grown men and women by irritating fluids and substances, such as wet sugar in the case of bakers and confectioners, and various color-stains in dye works. They seldom last for more than a few months, and usually narrow at their base and drop off, when the particular irritation that caused them ceases. On this account it is seldom worth while to try to remove them by burning with acids or cutting them off; and it is best not to pick at, or irritate, or scratch them too much.

CHAPTER XVII

THE PLUMBING AND SEWERING OF THE BODY

The Wastes of the Body. Almost everything that the body does in the process of living means the breaking down, or burning, of food; and produces, like every other kind of burning, two kinds of waste--"smoke" and "ashes."

The carbon dioxid "smoke," as we have already learned, is carried in the blood to the lungs, where it passes off in the breath. The solid part of our body waste, or the "ashes," is of two kinds--that which can be melted in water, or is, as we say, soluble; and that which cannot be melted in water, or is insoluble. The insoluble part of our solid body waste goes into the feces and is thus disposed of.

The soluble part of the body waste goes by a somewhat more roundabout route. With the carbon dioxid it is poured by the body cells into the veins, carried to the heart, and pumped through the lungs, where the carbon dioxid is thrown off. Going back to the heart it is pumped all over the body, part of it going through a very large artery to the liver, part through two large arteries to the kidneys, part to the skin, and the rest all over the remainder of the body.

The blood goes completely round the body-circuit from the heart to the fingers and toes, and back again to the heart, in less than forty-five seconds. Practically every drop of blood in the body will be pumped through the liver, the kidneys, and the skin, about once every half minute, so that they get plenty of chance to purify it thoroughly when they are working properly.

This sounds rather complicated; but is interesting, because it shows how much of a "mind of their own" the different organs and stuffs in our bodies have, or what, in scientific language, we call "power of selection." The skin glands pick out of the blood those waste substances which they are able to get rid of. The kidneys pick out another class of waste substances, which they are best able to deal with; while the liver which is the most important of all, attacks almost every kind of waste brought to it by the blood, and prepares it for disposal by the intestines, skin, and kidneys.

The Liver. The liver has a size to match its importance. It is the largest and heaviest gland, or organ, in the body, and weighs about three pounds, a little more than the brain. It buds off from the food tube just below the stomach, so that its waste tube, the bile duct--about the size of a goose quill--opens into the upper part of the intestine.

The main work of the liver is to receive the blood from all over the body and to act upon its waste substances, burning them up so that they can be taken up, and got rid of, by the glands of the skin and the kidneys. In the process it very frequently changes these waste substances from poisonous into harmless forms; and even when disease germs get into the body and infect it, the poisons, or toxins, which they pour into the blood are carried to the liver and there usually burned up, or turned into harmless substances.

The liver is, therefore, to be regarded as a great poison filter for the entire body. So long as it can deal with the poisons as fast as they are formed, either by the body itself, or in the food, or by disease germs, the body is safe and will remain healthy. But if the poisons come faster than the liver can deal with them, as, for instance, when we have eaten tainted meat or spoiled fruit, or have drunk alcohol, they begin to poison our nerves and muscles, and we become, as we say, "bilious." Our head aches, our tongue becomes coated, we have a bad taste in the mouth, we lose our appetite and feel stupid, dull, and feverish.

Such waste materials as the liver cannot burn down so that the kidneys and skin can handle them, it pours out through its duct into the intestine as the bile. The bile is a yellowish-brown fluid, which assists the pancreatic juice in the digestion of the food, and helps to dissolve the fats eaten, but is chiefly a waste product. It turns green when it has been acted upon by acids, or exposed to the air. So that the bile which you throw up when you are very sick at your stomach, is green because it has been acted upon by your gastric juice.

As you will remember, the blood which comes from the stomach and bowels is carried by the portal vein to the liver first and, through that, to the heart, instead of going directly to the heart, as all the other impure blood in the body does. This is owing, in part, to the fact that this blood, being full of substances freshly taken or made from the food, is very likely to contain poisons; indeed, as a matter of fact, blood taken from these veins on its way to the liver, and injected directly into the blood vessels of an animal, acts like a mild poison.

In part, however, this blood goes first to the liver, because the liver, besides being a great blood purifier, is a "blood-maker" in the sense that it changes raw food-stuffs in the blood from the intestines into forms which are more suitable for use by the brain, the muscles, and the other tissues of the body. Some of the sugars, for instance, the liver turns into a kind of animal starch (glycogen), which it stores away in its own cells. It also turns both sugars and proteins in the portal blood into fat, part of which it pours into the blood, and part of which it stores away also in its own cells. Thus the liver owes its great size partly to the large amount of blood-purifying, filtering, and poison-destroying work which it has to do, and partly to its acting as a storehouse of starch and fat, which the body can readily draw upon as it needs them.

As all poisons formed in, or entering, the body are brought to the liver for destruction, it is in an extremely exposed position, and very liable to break down under the attack of these poisons, whether of infectious diseases, or chloroform, or alcohol, or those formed by putrefaction in the stomach and intestines. This is why those who have lived long in the tropics and suffered from malaria, dysentery, and other infectious diseases, and those who drink too much alcohol, or have chronic indigestion, or dyspepsia, are likely to have swollen and inflamed livers.

The Gall Bladder. The liver has on its under side a little pear-shaped pouch called the gall bladder, in which the bile is stored before it is poured into the bowel. If this becomes inflamed by disease germs, or their poisons, in the blood, little hard masses will form inside it, usually about the size of a grain of corn, known as gall stones. So long as they stay in the gall bladder, they give little trouble, but if they start to pass out through the narrow bile duct into the intestine, they cause severe attacks of pain, known as "gall-stone colic," and, by blocking up the duct, may dam up the flow of the bile, force it back into the blood again, and stain all our tissues, including our skin and our eyes, yellow; and then we say we are jaundiced. Jaundice may also be caused by colds or other mild infections which attack the liver and bile ducts and clog the proper flow of the bile.

The Kidneys. The kidneys are another form of blood-filter, which deal chiefly with waste stuffs in the blood left from the proteins, or Meats, of our food-- meat, fish, milk, cheese, bread, peas, beans, etc. These waste-stuffs, called urea and urates, are formed in the liver and brought in the blood to the kidneys. These lie on either side of the backbone, opposite the small of the back, their lower ends being level with the highest point of the hip-bones, nearly six inches higher than they are usually supposed to be. When you think you have a "pain across the kidneys," it is usually a pain in the muscles of the back much lower down, and has nothing to do with the kidneys at all.

A very large artery carries the blood from the aorta to each side of the kidney, and a large vein carries the purified blood back to the vena cava and heart. Two smaller tubes about the size of a crow quill, the waste pipes of the kidneys (the ureters), carry the water containing urea and other waste substances strained out by the kidneys and called urine, down into a large pouch, the bladder, to be stored there until it can be got rid of.

The kidneys then are big filter-glands. They, like the lungs, are made up of a mesh, or network, of thousands of tiny tubes of two kinds, one set of tubes being blood vessels, and the other set the tiny branches of the kidney tubes which finally run together to form the ureters. The urine filters through from the spongy mesh of blood tubes (capillaries) into the kidney tubes and is poured out through the ureters. It is very important that the urine should be discharged as fast as it fills the bladder, that is, about once every three hours during the day. Nothing should be allowed to interfere with this; and whenever nature tells you that the bladder is full, it should be emptied promptly, or the poisons which nature is trying to get rid of in the urine may get back into the blood and cause serious trouble.

Diseases of the Kidneys. Naturally, the kidneys, working all the time and pouring out, as they do every day, from three to four pints of the liquid waste called urine, are subject to numerous diseases and disturbances. One of the common causes of these is failure to keep the skin thoroughly clean and healthy, as perspiration is of somewhat the same character as the urine; and if it be checked, it throws an extra amount of work upon the kidneys.

Another most important thing to keep the kidneys working well is to drink plenty of water, at least six or eight glasses a day, as well as to eat plenty of fresh green vegetables and fresh fruits, which, as we have seen, are eighty per cent water. Remember, we are a walking aquarium, and all our cells must be kept flooded with and soaked in water in order to be healthy. If the blood becomes overloaded with poisons, so much work may be thrown upon the kidneys that they will become inflamed and diseased and cannot form the urine properly; and then poisons accumulate in the system and finally produce serious illness and even death.

It was at one time believed that eating too much of certain kinds of foods, particularly those that leave much nitrogenous waste in the body, such as meat and fish, could produce a diseased condition of the kidneys, known as Bright's Disease; but we have found that the larger part of such cases are due to the attack of the germs of infectious diseases, particularly scarlet and typhoid fevers, tuberculosis, and colds. The popular impression that colds from wet feet or long drives in winter may "settle in the kidneys" is wrong, except in so far as those colds are caused by infectious germs.

Another cause of disturbance and permanent damage to the kidneys is the habitual use of alcohol. Even though this may be taken in only moderate amounts, the constant soaking of the tissues with even small amounts of alcohol may be most harmful to the kidneys, as well as to the liver.

CHAPTER XVIII

THE MUSCLES

Importance of the Muscles. It wouldn't be of much use to smell food, if we couldn't pick it up and bite it after we had reached it; or to see danger, if we were not able to move away from it. Every animal that lives, moves; and every movement, whether of the entire body from one place to another, or of parts of the body changing their relations to one another, or altering their shape, is carried out by an elastic, self-moving body-stuff, which we call muscle.

All the work that we do, whether in earning our living, or catching our food, or chewing it, or swallowing it and driving it through our food tube, or pumping the blood through our arteries, or drawing air into our lungs, is done by muscles. Hence, a very large part of the body has to be made of muscles. In fact, our muscles, put together, weigh almost as much as all the other stuffs in the body, making over forty per cent of our weight.

How the Muscles Act. The commonest form of muscle that we see is the red, lean meat of beef, mutton, or pork; and this will give us a good idea of how our own muscles look. All muscles, whatever their size or shape, are made up of little spindle-shaped or strap-shaped cells, or wriggling "body-cells" arranged in bands or strings. The size of a given muscle depends upon the number of cells that it contains.

The astonishing variety of movements which muscles can make is due to the fact that they have the power when stirred up, or stimulated, of changing their shape. As most of the muscle substance is arranged in bands, this change of shape on the part of the tiny cells that make up the band means that the band grows thicker and at the same time shorter,--just as a stretched rubber band does when it slackens,--so that it pulls nearer together the bones or other structures to which it is fastened at each end by fibrous cords called tendons, or sinews. This shortening of the muscle band is known as contraction.

When you wish, for instance, to lift your hand toward your face, you unconsciously send a message from your brain down the nerve cables in your spinal cord, out through the nerve-wires of your neck and shoulder, to the big biceps muscle on the front of your upper arm. This muscle then contracts, or shortens, and pulls up the forearm and hand, by bending the elbow joint. Just in proportion as the muscle becomes shorter, it becomes thicker in the middle; and this you can readily prove by grasping it lightly with your fingers when it contracts, and feeling it bulge.[22]

The food tube is surrounded with muscles, as you will remember, for moving the food along it, or churning it. These internal muscles, requiring only the presence of food to cause them to act, and not needing attention on the part of the brain or the will, are known as the involuntary ("without the will") muscles.

The great group of the voluntary, or bone-moving muscles, which move "with the will" and are under our direct control, may be divided roughly into two divisions--those that move the trunk, or body proper, and run, for the most part, lengthwise of it; and those that move the limbs.

On the body, they may be divided into two great sheets--one running up the front, and the other up the back. When those running up the front of the body contract, they naturally bend the back, and pull the head and shoulders forward and downward. Or, as when you spring up and catch the branch of a tree or a horizontal bar with your hands, these same muscles will pull the lower part of the body and legs upward, so that you can climb into the tree.

The largest and thickest bands of these front body muscles are found over the abdomen, or stomach, where you can feel them thicken and harden when you bend your body forward and pull with your arms, as in hauling on a rope. By their pressure upon the intestines, they give the bowels valuable support, assist in their movements, and help the circulation of the blood through them; so that it is of considerable importance to keep this entire group of muscles well toned up by exercises, such as swinging your arms back over your head, and then down between your legs; bending the head and shoulders backward and forward; swinging the legs up over the body, either when hanging from a bar or lying on your back. Proper exercising and toning up of these muscles will often cure constipation and dyspepsia, by their influence upon the bowels and stomach, and also keep one from taking on fat around the waist too rapidly.

On the back of the body, the muscle-sheet has grown into great, thick ropes of muscle on each side of the backbone, which you can feel hardening and softening in the small of the back, when you stoop down or lift weights. These are the muscles that hold the body erect, and keep the back straight when you stand, and are the largest and hardest working group of muscles in the body. Every minute that you sit, or stand, they are at work; and that is why they so often get tired out, and ache, and you say you have "a backache." They have to work harder to keep you erect or upright when you are standing perfectly still than when you walk or run, so that standing perfectly still is the hardest work you can do. Next to standing still, the hardest thing is to sit still, as you probably have found out. If it were not for these great muscles of the back and abdomen, we should double up like a jack-knife, either forward or backward, when we tried to stand up. It is not our skeleton that keeps us stiff or erect, but our muscles.

If you want to keep straight and erect, and thus have a good carriage, you must keep these great body muscles well trained and exercised by swinging movements, such as bending the back forward, standing with your feet apart and then swinging your head and shoulders down and between your legs; or, with your heels together, swinging your hands down till the fingers touch the ground; or by the different exercises that either bend your back, or hold it stiff and erect. Swinging from a bar, rowing, digging with a spade, chopping or sawing wood, dancing, rope-skipping, ball-playing, hop-scotch, and wrestling, all develop these muscles finely and are good for both boys and girls.

Other strands of these muscles branch out to fasten themselves to the shoulder blades and shoulders, where they help to draw the arm back as for a blow, pull the shoulders into position when you stand upright, or, when you have leaned forward and grasped something with the hand, help to pull up the arm and lift it from the ground. These muscles are quite important in holding the shoulders back and giving a good shape to the chest and good carriage of the upper part of the body and head. They are called into play in all exercises like striking, batting, tennis-playing, ball-throwing, swinging, shoveling, swimming, as well as in pulling, in lifting weights, in swinging an axe or handling a broom.

The muscles of the limbs are almost as numerous as those of the trunk of the body, and even more complex. Most of them, on both arms and legs, are in two great groups--one known as the "benders," or flexors, which, when they shorten, bend the limb; and the other, the "straighteners," or extensors, which straighten or extend it.

On the front of the arm, for instance, we have the large biceps ("two-headed") muscle, which runs from the shoulder to the bone of the forearm just below the elbow and, when it shortens, bends the elbow and lifts the arm toward the body.

On the back of the upper arm is the triceps ("three-headed") muscle, which is fastened at its lower end to a big spur of bone, the "point" of the elbow; when it shortens, acting lever fashion, it straightens or extends the arm. If this is done quickly, the fist is swung outward with force enough to strike quite a sharp blow, though, as you know, if you wish to hit really hard, you have to strike with the weight and muscles of the full arm and the body behind it, or, as we say, "from the shoulder."

In the lower limbs, the muscles are larger because they have heavier work to do, supporting and moving the whole weight of the body; but they are simpler in their arrangement since they have not such a variety of movements to carry out. The principal muscle in the thigh is the great muscle running down the front of the thigh, and fastening to the upper border of the patella, or knee cap. This muscle, when it shortens, straightens or extends the limb, or lifts the foot from the ground and swings it forward as in walking, or raises the knee up toward the body when we are sitting or lying down. You can easily tell how much it is used in walking by remembering how stiff and sore it gets when you have taken an unusually long tramp, particularly if there has been much hill-climbing in it. On the back of the thigh, runs another great group of muscles, which bend or flex the limb when they shorten. When the knee is bent, you can feel their tendons, or sinews, stand out as hard cords beneath the knee; hence, this group is called the ham-string muscles.[23]

How the Muscles are Fed. Our muscles are not only the largest, but the "livest" part of our bodies. Their contractions and movements are caused by their tiny "explosions" (like the chugging of an automobile, except that we can't hear them); and in this way they burn up the largest part of the food-fuel which we eat--mostly in the form of sugar. When they have burned up their surplus food-fuel, they call for more; and when this demand has been telegraphed to the brain, we say we are hungry, and that exercise has given us an appetite. While the muscles are at work, they demand that large supplies of fresh fuel shall be brought to them through the blood vessels; and this makes the heart beat harder and faster, and improves the circulation. As they burn up this fuel, they form smoke and ashes, or waste materials, which must be got rid of--the fluid part by perspiration from the surface of the skin, and through the kidneys, and the gas, or "smoke," through the lungs. This is the reason why, during exercise, we breathe faster and deeper than at other times, and why our skin begins first to glow and then to perspire.

If these waste-materials form in the muscles faster than the blood can wash them out, they poison the muscle-cells and we begin to feel tired, or fatigued. This is why our muscle-cells are often so stiff and sore next morning after a long tramp, or a hard day's work, or a football game. A hot bath or a good rub-down takes the soreness out of the muscles by helping them to get these poisonous wastes out of their cells.

Thus when we play or run or work, we are not only exercising our muscles and making them gain strength and skill, but we are stirring up, or stimulating, almost every part of our body to more vigorous and healthful action.

Indeed, as our muscles alone, of all our body stuffs, are under the control of the will, our only means of deliberately improving our appetites, or strengthening our hearts or circulation, or invigorating our lungs, or causing a large part of our brains and minds to grow and develop, is through muscular exercise. This is why nature has taken care to make us all so exceedingly fond of play, games, and sports of all sorts, in the open air, when we are young; and, as we grow older, to enjoy working hard and fighting and "hustling," as we say; and that is the reason, also, why we are now making muscular exercise such an important part of education.

FOOTNOTES:

[22] The muscle does not get any bigger when it contracts, as was at one time supposed; if you were to plunge it into a bath of water, and then cause it to contract, you would find that it did not raise the level of the water, showing that it was of exactly the same size as before, having lost as much in length as it gained in thickness.

[23] In the leg below the knee, and in the forearm, we have two groups of "benders" or flexors, and "straighteners" or extensors, as in the upper arm and leg, only slenderer and more numerous. They taper down into cord-like tendons at the wrist and ankle to fasten and to pull the hands and feet "open" and "shut," just as do the strings in the legs and arms of a puppet or mechanical doll, or the sinews in the foot of a chicken.

CHAPTER XIX

THE STIFFENING RODS OF THE BODY-MACHINE

What Bones Are. The bones are not the solid foundation and framework upon which the body is built, as they are usually described. They are simply a framework of rods and plates which "petrified," or turned into spongy limestone after the body was built, to make it firmer and stiffen it for movement. All the animals below the fishes, such as worms, sea-anemones, oysters, clams, and insects, get along very well without any bones at all; and when we are born, our bones, which haven't fully "set" yet, are still gristly and soft. The cores of the limbs, as they begin to stiffen, first turn into gristle, or cartilage, and later into bone; indeed, many of our bones remain gristle in parts until we are fifteen or sixteen years of age. This is why children's bones, being softer and more flexible than those of grown-up people, are not so liable to break or snap across when they fall or tumble about; and why, too, they are more easily warped or bent out of shape through lack of proper muscular exercise and proper food.

Bones are strips of soft body-stuff soaked with lime and hardened, like bricklayer's mortar, or concrete.[24] When you know the shape of the body, you know the bones; for they simply form a shell over the head and run like cores, or piths, down the centre of the back, and down each joint of the limbs.

In turning into spongy limestone, or animal concrete, they have become one of the deadest tissues in the body. They are tools of the muscles, the levers by which the muscles move the limbs and body about; they never do anything of their own accord. On account of their lifelessness and lack of vitality, they are rather easily attacked by disease, or broken by a blow or fall. There are such a large number of bones (two hundred and six, all told), and they resist decay and last so much longer after death than any other parts of the body, that they fill our museums and text-books of anatomy, form most of our fossils, and have thus given us rather an exaggerated idea of their importance during life.

The Frame-Work of the Body. Just look at any part of the body and imagine that it has a bony core of about the same general shape as itself, and you can reason out all the bones of the skeleton. To begin at the top, the skull is a box of strong, plate-like bones, which have hardened to protect the brain as it grew; and the shape of its upper, or brain, part is exactly that of the head, as you can easily feel by laying your hands upon it. Then come bony shells, or sockets, for the eyes and nose; and, below these, two heavy half-circles of bone, like the jaws of a steel trap, to carry the teeth.

The thickness of the lower jaw and the size and squareness of the angle where it bends upward to be hinged to the skull, below the ear, are what give the appearance of squareness and determination to the faces of strong, vigorous men or women. If we want to imply that a person has a feeble will, or weak character, we say he has a "weak jaw."

The skull rests upon the top of the backbone, or spinal column, which, instead of being one long solid bone, is made up of a number of pieces, or sections, known as vertebr? Each one of these vertebr?has a ring, or arch, upon its back. These, running one after the other, form a jointed, bony tube to protect the spinal cord, or main nerve-cable of the body, which runs through it.

Although the backbone can bend forward or backward, or twist from side to side a little, by the little pieces of bone of which it is built up gliding and turning upon one another, it is really very stiff and rigid, so as to protect the spinal cord and prevent its being stretched or pinched. Most of the movements which we call bending the spine are really movements of other joints which connect the body or head with it. When we bend our necks, for instance, we hardly bend the backbone at all, as most of the movement is made in the joint at the top of it, between it and the skull. Similarly, when we bend our backs, we really bend our backbones very little; for most of the movement comes at the hip joints, between the thighs and the hip bones.

Each of the limbs has a single, long, rounded bone in the upper part, known in the arm as the humerus, and two bones in the lower part. These last are known as the radius and ulna (the "funny bone") in the forearm, and the tibia and fibula in the leg. The shoulder-joint is made by the rounded head of the humerus fitting into the shallow cup of the scapula, or shoulder-blade. It is shallower than the hip joint to allow it freer movement; but this makes it weaker and much more easily dislocated, or put out of joint,--the most so, in fact, of any joint in the body.

The hip joints are deep, strong, cup-shaped sockets upon each side of the hip bones, or pelvis, into which fit the heads of the femurs or thigh bones. When the hip joint does become dislocated, it is very hard to put back again, on account of its depth and the heavy muscles surrounding it. It is quite subject to the attack of tuberculosis, or "hip-joint disease."

The joints, or points at which the bones join one another, look rather complicated, but they are really as simple as the bones themselves. Each joint has practically made itself by the two bones' rubbing against each other, until finally their ends became moulded to each other, and formed the ball-and-socket, or the hinge, according to whichever the movements of the "bend" required. The ends, or heads, of the bones which form a joint are covered with a smooth, shining coating of cartilage, or gristle, so that they glide easily over each other.

Around each joint has grown up a strong sheath of tough, fibrous tissue to hold the bones together; and, inside this, between the heads of the bones, is a very delicate little bag, or pouch, containing a few drops of smooth, slippery fluid (synovial fluid) to lubricate the movements of the joint. This is sometimes called the "joint oil," though it is not really oil.

Bones are covered with a tough skin, or membrane (periosteum). They are hardest and most solid on their surfaces, and hollow, or spongy, inside. The long bones of the limbs are hollow, and the cavity is filled with a delicate fat called marrow--just as an elderberry stem or willow-twig is filled with pith. This tubular shape makes them as strong as if they were solid, and much lighter.[25]

The short, square, and flattened bones of the body, such as those of the wrist, the skull, and the hips, instead of being hollow inside are spongy; and the spaces in the bone-sponge are filled with a soft tissue called the red marrow in which new red and white corpuscles for the blood are born, to take the place of those which die and go to pieces.

FOOTNOTES:

[24] You can easily prove that a bone is made up of living tissue soaked and stiffened with lime, by putting it into a jar filled with weak acid. This will gradually dissolve and melt out the lime salts, and then you will find that the bone has lost three-fourths of its weight and that what remains of it is so soft and flexible that it can be bent, or even tied into a knot.

[25] The hollow spaces in the bones of birds, however, are filled with air, which makes them lighter for flying.

CHAPTER XX

OUR TELEPHONE EXCHANGE AND ITS CABLES

The Brain. We are exceedingly proud of our brain and inclined to regard it as the most important part of our body. So it is, in a sense; for it is the part which, through its connecting wires, called the nerves, ties together all the widely separated organs and regions in our body, and helps them to work in harmony with one another. We speak of it as the master and controller of the body; but this is only partially true.

The brain is not so much the President of our Cell Republic as a great central telephone exchange, where messages from all over the body are received, sifted, and transmitted in more or less modified form, to other parts of the body. Three-fourths of the work of the brain consists in acting as "middle-man," or transmitter, of messages from one part of the body to another. In fact, the brain is far more the servant of the body than its ruler; and depends for its food supply, its protection, its health, and its very life, upon the rest of the body. The best way to keep the brain clear and vigorous is to keep the muscles of the stomach, the liver, the heart, and the entire body in good health.

What the Brain Does. The brain is the very wonderful organ with which we do what we are pleased to call our thinking, and also a number of other more important things of which we are not conscious at all. It is a large organ, weighing nearly three pounds when full grown. In shape it is like an oval loaf of bread split lengthwise by a great groove down the centre, and with a curiously wrinkled or folded surface. The two halves of the brain, called hemispheres (though more nearly the shape of a coffee-bean), are alike; and each one, by some curious twist, or freak, of nature, receives messages from, and controls, the opposite half of the body--the right half controlling the left side of the body, while the left half controls the right side of the body. Thus an injury or a hemorrhage on the left side of the brain will produce paralysis of the right side, which is the side on which a stroke of paralysis most commonly occurs.

All the nerve fibres in each half or hemisphere of the upper brain run downward and inward like the sticks of a fan, to meet in a strap-like band, or stalk, which connects it with the base of the brain and the spinal cord. A very small amount of damage at this central part, or base, of the brain will produce a very large amount of paralysis. We may have large pieces of the bones of the skull driven into the outer surface of the brain, or considerable masses of our upper brain removed, or destroyed by tumors or disease, without very serious injury. But any disease or injury which falls upon the base of the brain, where these stalks run and big nerve-knots (ganglia) lie, will cause very serious damage, and often death.

The whole upper brain is a department of superintendence, which has grown up from the lower brain to receive messages, compare them with each other, and with the records of previous messages which it has stored up, thus giving us the powers which we call memory, judgment, and thought. Unfortunately, however, long and carefully as we have studied the brain, we really know little about the way in which it carries out these most important processes of memory, of judgment, and of thought, or even of the particular parts of it in which each of these is carried out.

No part of the brain, for instance, seems to be specially devoted to, or concerned in, memory or reason or imagination, still less to any of the emotions, such as anger, joy, jealousy or fear; so all those systems which pretend to tell anything about our mental powers and our dispositions by feeling the shapes of our heads, or the bumps on them, are pure nonsense.

The most important and highest part of the brain is its surface, a thin layer of gray nerve-stuff, often spoken of as the gray matter (the cortex, or "bark"), which is thrown into curious folds, or wrinkles, called convolutions. This gray matter is found in the parts of the nervous system where the most important and delicate work is done. The rest of the nervous system is made up of what is called white matter, from its lighter color; and this is chiefly mere bundles of telephone wires carrying messages from one piece of gray matter to another, or to the muscles.

We also know that a certain rather small strip of the upper brain-surface, or cortex, about the size of two fingers, running upward and backward from just above the ear, controls the movements of the different parts of the body. One little patch of it for the hand, another for the wrist, another for the arm, another for the shoulder, another for the foot, and so on. We can even pick out the little patch which controls so small a part of the body as the thumb or the eyelids. So when we have a tumor of the brain or an injury to the skull in this region, we can tell, by noticing what groups of muscles are paralyzed, almost exactly where that injury or tumor is. Then we can drill a hole in the skull directly over it and remove the tumor, lift up the splinter of bone, or tie the ruptured blood vessel.

Three other patches, or areas, running along the side of the brain, each of them about two inches across, are known to be the centres for smell, hearing, and sight, that for sight lying furthest back. Damage to one of these areas will make the individual more or less completely blind, or deaf, or deprived of the sense of smell, as the case may be.

At the lower part of the area which controls the muscles of the different parts of the body, above and a little in front of the tip of the ear, lies a very important centre, which controls the movements of the tongue and lips, and is known as the speech centre. If this should be injured or destroyed, the power of speech is entirely lost. This, curiously enough, lies upon the left side of the brain, and is the only one-sided centre in the body. Why this is so is somewhat puzzling, except that as speech is made up both of sound and of gesture, and our gestures are usually made with the right hand, it is not unreasonable to suppose that the speech centre should have grown up on that side of the brain which controls the right hand, which is, as you remember, the left hemisphere. What makes this more probable is that in persons who are "left-handed," the speech centre lies upon the opposite or right side of the brain. So it is waste of time and does more harm than good to try to "break" any child of left-handedness.

The Spinal Cord. Running downward from the base of the brain, like the stalk of a flower, is a great bundle of nerve-fibres, the central cable of our body telephone system, the spinal cord. This, you will remember, runs through a bony tube formed by the arches of the successive vertebrae; and as it runs down the body, like every other cable it gives off and receives branches connecting it with the different parts of the body through which it passes. These branches are given off in pairs, and run out through openings between the little sections of bone, or vertebrae, of which the spinal column is made up. They are called the spinal nerves, and each pair supplies the part of the body which lies near the place where it comes out of the cord.

The spinal nerves contain nerve wires of two sorts--the inward, or sensory, and the outward, or motor, nerves. The sensory, or ingoing, nerves come from the muscles and the skin and bring messages of heat and cold, of touch and pressure, of pain and comfort, to the spinal cord and brain. The outward, or motor, nerves running in the same bundle go to the muscles and end in curious little plates on the surface of the tiny muscle fibres, and carry messages from the spinal cord and brain, telling the muscles when and how to contract.

As the spinal cord runs down the body, it becomes gradually smaller, as more and more branches are given off, until finally, just below the small of the back and opposite the hip bones, it breaks up by dividing into a number of large branches which go to supply the hips and lower limbs.

While most of the spinal cord is made up of bundles of white fibres, carrying messages from the body to the brain, its central portion, or core, is made of gray matter. The reason for this is that many of the simpler messages from the surface of the body and the movements that they require are attended to by this gray matter, or ganglia, of the spinal cord without troubling the brain at all.

For instance, if you were sound asleep, and somebody were to tickle the sole of your bare foot very gently, the nerves of the skin would carry the message to the gray matter of the spinal cord, and it would promptly order the muscles of the leg to contract, and your foot would be drawn away from the tickling finger, without your brain taking any part in the matter, though, if you had been awake, you would of course have known what was going on.

This sort of reply to a stimulus, or "stirring up," without our knowing anything about it, is known as a reflex movement. Not only are many of these reflexes carried out without any help from the will, or brain, but they are so prompt and powerful that the brain, or will, can hardly stop them if it tries, as, for instance, in the case of tickling the feet. You can, if you make up your mind to it, prevent yourself from either wriggling, pulling your foot away, or giggling, when the sole of your foot is tickled; but if you happen to be at all "ticklish," it will take all the determination you have to do it, and some children are utterly unable to resist this impulse to squirm when tickled.

This extraordinary power of your reflexes has developed because only the promptest possible response, by jerking your hand away or jumping, will be quick enough to save your life in some accidents or emergencies, when it would take entirely too long to telephone up to the brain and get its decision before jumping. When you are badly frightened, you often jump first and discover that you are frightened afterwards; and this jump, under certain circumstances, may save your life. On the other hand, like all instinctive or impulsive movements, it may get you into more trouble than if you had kept still.

As you will see by the picture, the spinal nerves, which are given off from the cord in the lower part of the neck and between the shoulder blades, are gathered together into a great loose bundle to form the long nerve-wires needed to supply the shoulders and arms. Those given off from the small of the back just above the hips also run together to form, first a network and then a big single nerve-cord, called the sciatic nerve, which many of you have probably heard of from the frightfully painful disease due to an inflammation of it, called sciatica. It is the largest nerve-cord in the body, running down the middle of the back of the thigh to supply the muscles of two-thirds of the leg.[26]

The substance of both the spinal cord and the brain is made up of millions of delicate, tiny cells, called neurons, most of which, with very long branches, are arranged in chains for carrying messages, forming the white matter; while the others lie in groups, or ganglia, for sorting and deciding upon messages, forming the gray matter.

Just at the top of the spinal cord, where it passes into the skull and joins with the brain, it swells out into a sort of knob, about the size of a queen olive or the head of a gold-headed cane, which is known as the medulla, or "pith." This is the most vital single part of the entire brain and nervous system; and the smallest direct injury to it will produce instant death, partly because all the messages which pass between the brain and the body have to go through it, and partly because in it are situated the centres which control breathing and the beat of the heart, and another quite important but less vital centre,-- that for swallowing.

How Messages are Received and Sent. Now to learn how smoothly and beautifully this nerve telephone system of ours works, and how simple it really is, although it has such a large number of lines and so many telephones on each line, and such a large central exchange, let us see how it deals with a message from the outside world. Suppose you are running barefoot and step on a thorn. Instantly the tiny nerve bulbs in the skin of the sole of your foot are stimulated, or set in vibration, and they send these vibrations up the sciatic nerve, into and up the whole length of the spinal cord, through the medulla, which switches them over to the other side of the brain up through the brain stalk, and out to the part of the surface (cortex) of the brain which controls the movements of the foot. All this takes only a fraction of a second, but it is not until the message reaches the brain-surface that you feel pain. If you were to cut the sciatic nerve, or even tie a string tightly around it, you could prick or burn the sole of your foot as much as you pleased, and you would not feel any pain at all.

As soon as the surface of the brain has recognized the pain and where it comes from, it promptly sends a return message back down the same cable, though by different nerve-wires, to the muscles of the foot and leg, saying, "Jerk that foot away!" As a matter of fact, this message will arrive too late, for the centres in the spinal cord will already have attended to this part of the matter, often almost before you know that you are hurt.

However, there is plenty of other work for the brain to do; and its next step, quicker than you can think, is to wake up a dozen muscles all over the body with the order, "Sit down!" And you promptly sit down. At the same time, the brain "central" has ordered the muscles of your arms and hands to reach down and pick up the foot, partly to protect it from any further scratch, and partly to pull the thorn out of it. Next it rushes a hurry call to the muscles controlling your lungs and throat, and says, "Howl!" and you howl accordingly. Another jab at the switchboard, and the eyes are called up and ordered to weep, while at the same time the muscles of the trunk of your body are set in rhythmic movement by another message, and you rock yourself backward and forward.

This weeping and rocking yourself backward and forward and nursing your foot seem rather foolish,--indeed you have perhaps often been told that they are both foolish and babyish,--but, as you say, you "can't help it," and there is a good reason for it. The howl is a call for help; and if the hurt were due to the bite of a wolf or a bear, or the cut had gone deep enough to open an artery, this dreadfully unmusical noise might be the means of saving your life; while the rocking backward and forward and jerking yourself about would also send a message that you needed help, supposing you were so badly hurt that you couldn't call out, to anyone who happened to be within sight of you. So that it isn't entirely babyish and foolish to howl and squirm about when you are hurt--though it is manly to keep both within reasonable limits.

If the message about the thorn had been brought by your eyes,--in other words, if you had seen it before you stepped on it,--then a similar but much simpler and less painful reflex would have been carried out. The image of the thorn would fall on the retina of the eye and through its optic nerve the message would be flashed to the brain: "There is something slim and sharp in the path,--looks like a thorn." When this message reached the brain, and not till then, would you see the thorn, just as in the case of the pain message from the foot. Then the brain would take charge of the situation just as before, flashing a hasty message to the muscles of the legs, saying, "Jump!" while its message to the throat and lungs, instead of "Yell," would be merely, "Say, 'Goodness!' or 'Whew!'" and you would say it and run on.

If the thing in the grass, instead of a thorn, happened to be a snake, and you heard it rustle, then the warning message would come through your ears to the brain, and you would jump just the same; though, as it is not so easy to tell by a hearing message exactly where the sound is coming from, you might possibly jump in the wrong direction and land on top of the danger.

This is the way in which you see, hear, and form ideas of things. Your eye telegraphs to the brain the colors; your ear, the sounds; and your nose, the smells of the particular object; and then your brain puts these all together and compares them with its records of things that it has seen before, which looked, or sounded, or smelt like that, and decides what it is; and you say you see an apple, or you hear a rooster crow, or you smell pies baking. Remember that, strange as it may seem, you don't see an orange, for instance, but only a circular patch of yellowness, which, when you had seen it before, and felt of it with your hand, you found to be associated with a feeling of roundness and solidness; and when you lifted it toward your nose, with the well-known smell of orange-peel; so you called it an orange. If the yellow patch were hard, instead of elastic, to the touch, and didn't have any aromatic smell when you brought it up to your nose, you would probably say it was a gourd, or an apple, or perhaps a yellow croquet ball. This is the way in which, we say, our senses may "deceive" us, and is one of the reasons why three different people who have seen something happen will often differ so much in their accounts of it.

It is not so much that our senses deceive us, but that we draw the wrong conclusions from the sights, sounds, and smells that they report to our brains, usually from being in too great a hurry and not looking carefully enough, or not waiting to check up what we see by touching, hearing, or tasting the thing that we look at.

This message-and-answer system runs all through our body. For instance, if we run fast, then the muscle cells in our legs burn up a good deal of sugar-fuel, and throw the waste gas, or smoke, into the blood. This is pumped by the heart all over the body, in a few seconds. When this carbon dioxid reaches the breathing centre in the medulla, it stirs it up to send promptly a message to the lungs to breathe faster and deeper, while, at the same time, it calls upon the circulation centre close to it, to stir up the heart and make it beat harder and faster, so as to give the muscles more blood to work with. If some poisonous or very irritating food is swallowed, as soon as it begins to hurt the cells lining the stomach, these promptly telegraph to the vomiting centre in the brain, we begin to feel "sick at the stomach," the brain sends the necessary directions to the great muscles of the abdomen and the diaphragm, they squeeze down upon the stomach, and its contents are promptly pumped back up the gullet and out through the mouth, thus throwing up the poisons.

And so on all over the body--every tiniest region or organ in the body, every square inch of the skin, has its special wire connecting it with the great telephone exchange, enabling it to report danger, and to call for help or assistance the moment it needs it.

FOOTNOTES:

[26] To give you an idea of what real things nerve-trunks are, this sciatic nerve is as large as a small clothes-line, or, more accurately, as a carpenter's lead pencil, and so strong that when the surgeon cuts down upon it and stretches it to cure a very bad case of sciatica, he can lift the lower half of the body clear of the table by it. This strength, of course, is not due to the nerve-fibres and cells themselves but to the tough, fibrous sheath, or covering, with which all the nerves that run outside of the brain and spinal cord are covered

and coated. The spinal cord, though it is between one-half and three-fourths of an inch across, or about the size of an ordinary blackboard pointer, has little or none of this fibrous tissue in it, and is very soft and delicate, easily torn when its bony case is broken; hence its old name, the spinal marrow, from its apparent resemblance to the marrow, or soft fat, in the hollow of a bone.

CHAPTER XXI

THE HYGIENE OF BONES, NERVES, AND MUSCLES

HOW TO GET AND KEEP A GOOD FIGURE

Erect Position is the Result of Vigorous Health. Naturally and properly, an erect, graceful figure and a good carriage have always been keenly desired; and much attention has been paid to the best means of acquiring them; as we say, we try to "get the habit" of carrying ourselves straight and well. But it must be remembered that an erect figure and a good carriage are the results of health and vigor, rather than the cause of them.

Stooping, round shoulders, sitting "all hunched up," or a shuffling gait, are owing partly to bad habits, or "slouchiness," but chiefly to weak muscles and a badly-fed nervous system, often due to a poor digestion and a weak circulation. If a child is not healthy and vigorous, then no amount of drilling or reminders to "sit straight" and "stand erect" will make him do so.

It is of great importance that the child should take an erect and correct position for reading and writing, and while sitting at his desk; and that the desk and the seat should fit him. But it is more important that he should not sit at his desk in a stuffy room long enough to be harmed by a cramped position.

There are few children who will "hump over" at their desks, if the muscles of their backs and necks are strong and vigorous, and their brains well ventilated. Nor will many of them bore their noses into their books, or sprawl all over their copy books when they write, unless the light is poor, or they have some defect of the eyes which has not been corrected by proper glasses. A bad position or a bad carriage in a child is a sign of ill health, and should be treated by the removal of its cause.

Curvatures--Their Cause and Cure. There are various forms of curvatures, or bendings, of the spine which are supposed to be owing to faulty positions of sitting or of carrying the body. There is wide difference of opinions as to their cause; but this all are agreed on, that they practically never occur in sturdy, well-grown, active children; and the way that they are now corrected is by careful systems of balancing, muscular exercise, open-air life, and abundant feeding, instead of using steel braces, or jackets, or schoolroom drills.

Much the same is true of other deformities and defects of the body, as, for instance, round shoulders, or "flat-foot," or even such serious ones as "club-foot" and "bow-legs." Nearly all these are caused by the weakness or wrong action of some muscle, or groups of muscles. If this be long continued or neglected, the bones--which, you will remember, were made by the muscles in the first place--will be warped out of shape. When this has occurred, it is often necessary to bring back the limb, or foot, into a nearly straight position by mechanical or surgical means; but we now largely depend upon muscular exercises combined with rubbing and massage with the hand, and on building up the general vigor of the entire body, so that the muscles will pull the limb or the backbone back into proper position. Take care of the muscles, and the bones will take care of themselves! Make the body strong, vigorous, and happy, and it will "hold" and "carry" itself.

OUR FEET

The Living Arches of the Foot. One of the most important things to look after, if we wish to have an erect carriage and a swift, graceful gait, is the shape and vigor of the feet. Each foot consists of two springy, living arches of bone and sinew, which are also used as levers, one running lengthwise from the heel to the ball of the toes, and the other crosswise at the instep. These arches are built largely of bones, but are given that springy, elastic curve on which their health and comfort depend, and are kept in proper shape and position, solely by the action of muscles--those of the lower part of the leg and calf.

The absence of impression on the inner border of the normal footprint at A is due to the elevation of the foot by the longitudinal arch. The other arch lies across the foot in front of this.--After Schmidt.]

The purpose of these arches is to "give," or spring, like carriage springs, and thus break the shock of each step and cause the body to "ride" easily and comfortably. In order that a spring may "give," it must expand, or spread. Far the commonest and most serious cause of a poor, easily tired gait and a bad carriage is tight shoes, which, by being too short, or too narrow, or both, prevent the arches of the foot from "giving" and expanding. Not only does this produce corns, bunions, and lame feet, but it makes both standing and walking painful and feeble, and destroys the balance of the entire body, causing the back to ache, the shoulders to droop forward, and the neck muscles to tire themselves out trying to pull the head back so as to keep the face and eyes erect. Thus one soon tires, and never really enjoys walking. If this disturbance of balance is increased by high heels, thrust forward under the middle of the foot, the result is very bad.

(1) A foot that has never worn a shoe (from a photograph); (2) A foot so cramped and bent as to prevent firmness of step and gait.]

Our Shoes, an Important Factor in Health. Few more ingenious instruments of crippling and torture have ever been invented than fashionable tight shoes with high heels.

Kipling never said a shrewder or truer thing than when he made Mulvaney, the old Irish drill-sergeant, tell the new recruit, "Remimber, me son, a soljer on the marrch is no betther than his feet!" and this applies largely to the march of life as well.

Every shoe should be at least three-quarters of an inch longer, and from half to three-quarters of an inch wider, than the foot at rest, to allow proper expansion of these great "carriage-spring" arches. If children run free in the open air, either barefoot, or with light, loose, well-ventilated shoes, or sandals, they will have little trouble, not only with bunions, corns, "flat-foot," or lameness, but also with their backs, their gait, and their carriage. Easily half of our backaches, and inability to walk far or run fast in later life, to say nothing of over-fatness and dyspepsia, are caused by tight shoes.

SLEEP AND REST

Why We Need Rest. A most important element in a life of healthful exercise, study, and play is rest. Even when we are hard at work, we need frequent breathing spells and changes of occupation and amusement to keep one part of our muscles, or our brains, from poisoning itself. But after a time, in even the strongest and toughest of us, there comes a period when no change of occupation, no mere sitting still, will rest us; we begin to feel drowsy and want to go to sleep. This means partly that the fatigue poisons, in spite of fresh air and change, have piled up faster than we can burn them, so that we need sleep to restore the body.

All day long we are making more carbon dioxid than the oxygen we breathe in can take care of; while we sleep, the situation is reversed--the oxygen is gaining on the carbon dioxid. This is why the air in our bedrooms ought to be kept especially pure and fresh.

But the need goes deeper than this: sleeping and waking are simply parts of the great rhythm in which all life beats--a period of work followed by a period of rest. Continuous, never-ceasing activity for any living thing quickly means death. While externally the body appears to be at rest, the processes of growth and upbuilding probably go on more rapidly when we are asleep than when we are awake. The benefits of exercise are made permanent and built into the body during the sleep that follows it. The more rapidly young animals are growing, the more hours out of the twenty-four they spend in sleep. When you sleep, you are not stopping all the useful activities of your body and mind, you are simply giving some of the most useful and most important of them a chance to work. The only likeness between sleep and death is that in both the body is quiet and the eyes are closed. Really we are never more alive and growing than when asleep.

It is of the utmost importance that young children especially have all the sleep they need, and that is precisely all that they can be induced to take. The best rule for you, then, to follow, is to go to bed when you feel sleepy, and to get up when you wake rested. Every child under twelve should have at least ten hours of sleep, and every grown person eight, or better still, nine hours. Time spent in sound, refreshing sleep, is time well spent. If you cannot sleep well, it is a signal that something is wrong with your health, or your habits--a danger signal of great importance, which should be attended to at once. The best and only safe sleep-producer is exercise in the open air.

DISORDERS OF MUSCLES AND BONES

The Muscles and Bones Have Few Diseases. Considering how complex it is, and the never-ceasing strain upon it, this moving apparatus of ours, the nerve-bone-muscle-machine, is surprisingly free from disease. The muscles, though they form nearly half our bulk, have scarcely a single disease peculiar to them, or chiefly beginning in them, unless fatigue and its consequences might be so regarded. They may become weakened and wasted by either lack or excess of exercise, by under-feeding, or by loss of sleep; but most of their disturbances are due to poisons which have got into the blood pumped through them, or to paralysis or other injuries to the nerves that supply them.

The muscles of an arm, for instance, which has been lashed to a splint, or shut tightly in a cast for a long time, waste away and shrink until the arm becomes, as we say, "just skin and bone"; and the same thing will happen if the nerve supplying a muscle, or a limb, is cut or paralyzed.

The bones have more diseases than the muscles, but really comparatively few, considering their great number and size, and the constant strain to which they are subjected in supporting the body, and driving it forward and doing its work under the handling and leverage of the muscles. Most of their diseases are, like those of the muscles, the after-effects of general diseases, particularly the infections and fevers, which begin elsewhere in the body; and the best treatment of such bone diseases is the cure and removal of the disease that caused them.

Repair of Broken Bones. If bones are broken by a fall, or blow, they display a remarkable power of repair. The "skin" covering them (periosteum) pours out a quantity of living lime-cement, or animal-mortar, around the two broken ends, which solders them together, much as a plumber will make a joint between the ends of two pipes. This repair substance is called callus. The most remarkable thing about the process is that, when it has held the two broken ends together long enough for them to "knit" firmly--that is, to connect their blood vessels and marrow cavities properly--this handful of lime-cement, which has piled up around the break, gradually melts away and disappears; so that, if the ends of the bone have been brought accurately together, you can hardly tell where the break was, except by a slight ridge or thickening.

TROUBLES OF THE NERVOUS SYSTEM

The Nervous System is not easily Damaged. The nervous system is subject to a good many more diseases than are either the muscles or the bones; but, considering how complex it is, it is not nearly so easily damaged or thrown out of balance as we usually imagine, and has astonishing powers of repair. Instead of being one of the first parts of the body to be attacked by a disease, such as an infection or a fever, it is one of the very last to feel the effects of disease, except in the sense that it often gives early that invaluable danger signal, pain.

Headache. Next after fatigue the most valuable danger signal given us by our nerves is that commonest of all pains, headache. Indeed, it is not too much to say that headache is the most useful pain in the world. It has little to do with the condition of the brain, but occurs in the head chiefly because the nerves of the head and face are the most sensitive of all those in the body, and the first ones, therefore, to "cry out" when hurt.

Headache has been described as the cry of a poisoned or starved or over-worked nerve, and is simply nature's signal that something is going wrong. Toxins, or poisons, formed anywhere in the body, from any cause, get into the blood, are carried to the sensitive nerves of the head and face, and irritate them so that they ache. It is foolish to try to do anything to the head itself for the relief of headache, although cold cloths, or a hot-water bottle, may be soothing in mild cases. The thing to do is to clear the poison out of the blood, and the only way is to find what has caused it.

Nearly all the things that cause headache do so by poisoning the blood. A very common cause of headache, for instance, is getting over-tired, especially if at the same time you do not get enough sleep; and, as you already know, tiredness, or fatigue, is a form of self-poisoning. Another very common cause of headache is bad air--sitting or sleeping in hot, stuffy rooms with the windows shut tight. If you do this, not only are you not getting oxygen enough into your blood to burn up the waste poisons that your own cells are making all the time, but also you are breathing in the waste poisons from other people's lungs, and the germs that are always in bad air.

Another very common cause of headache is eye-strain. Whenever you find that, when you try to read, the letters begin to dance before your eyes, and your head soon begins to ache, it is a sign that you need to have your eyes examined and perhaps a pair of glasses fitted to enable you to see properly.

Constipation and disturbances of digestion also very often cause headache by poisoning the blood; and, as you know, the first sign of a bad cold, or the beginning of a fever, or other illness, will often be a bad headache.

In short, a headache always means that something is going wrong; and the thing to do is to set to work at once to see if you can find out what has caused it, and then to remove the cause. If you cannot find out the cause, then go to a doctor and ask him to tell you what it is, and what to do to get rid of it.

Above all things, don't swallow a dose of some kind of headache medicine, and go on with your work, or your bad habits of eating, or using your eyes; because, even though it may relieve the pain, it doesn't do anything whatever to remove the cause and leaves you just as badly off as you were before you took it. Besides, most of these headache medicines, which for a time will relieve the pain of a headache, are narcotics, or pain-deadeners; and in more than very moderate doses they are poisons, and often dangerous ones. Those in commonest use, known as the "coal tar" remedies, because the chemists make them out of coal tar,[27] are likely to have a weakening effect upon the heart; and, while not very dangerous in small doses, they are very bad things to get into the habit of using.

The Exaggerated Claims of Patent Medicines. The same thing must be said of the habit of dosing yourself every time you feel a pain or an ache, with some sort of medicine, whether obtained at some previous time from a doctor, or bought at a drug store. A large majority of the medicines that are most widely advertised to cure all sorts of pains and aches contain some form of narcotic-- most commonly either alcohol or opium. The reason for this is that no one medicine can possibly be a cure for all sorts of diseases; and the only kind of medicine that will make almost every one who takes it feel a little bit better for the time being is a narcotic, because it has the power of deadening the nerves to pain or discomfort.

Careful analyses by boards of health and government chemists of a great number of advertised medicines have shown that three-fourths of the so-called tonics and "bitters" and "bracers" of all sorts contain alcohol--some of them in such large amounts as to be stronger and more intoxicating than whiskey. The same investigations have found that a large majority of the "colic cures," "pain relievers," nearly all the "soothing syrups" and "teething syrups," and most of the cough mixtures, cough cures, and consumption cures contain opium, often in quite dangerous amounts. The widely-advertised medicines and remedies guaranteed to cure all sorts of diseases in a very short time are almost certain to be one of two things: either out-and-out frauds, costing about four cents a bottle and selling for fifty cents or a dollar, or else dangerous poisons. All patent pain relievers are safe things to let entirely alone.

Another risk in taking medicines wholesale, especially those that are known as patent medicines, is that you never can be quite sure what you are taking, as their composition is usually kept a strict secret. It may happen to be something very good for your disease, it may be entirely useless, and it may be something very harmful. There is no one drug, or medicine, known to the medical profession, that will cure more than one or two diseases, or relieve more than four or five disturbed and uncomfortable conditions. As you not only do not know what you are taking, but are not always quite sure what is the matter with you, the chances of your getting the right remedy for your disease are not much more than one in a hundred. If it isn't the right thing, you are certainly wasting your money, and may be doing yourself a serious injury.

We should not pour drugs of which we know little into a body of which we know less. Doctors give scarcely a fourth as much medicine now as they did fifty years ago. The best cures are food, exercise, sleep, and fresh air.

The Effects of Disease. In the case of nearly all infectious diseases, the effects on the nervous system are among the last to appear, and may not occur until weeks, months, or even years after the main fever or attack of sickness. This is one of the reasons why, when they do occur, they are often hard to cure; the whole system has become saturated with the poisons before they reach the nerves at all. So it happens that the idea has grown up that nervous diseases are very hard to cure. When, however, we know that two-thirds of them are a late result of some of the preventable infectious diseases and fevers, we can realize that it is perfectly possible to prevent them, and that prevention is the best cure.

The poisons that attack the brain and nervous system may be formed in the body by disease germs or brought in from without, as are alcohol, tobacco, lead, or arsenic. Even such mild infections as measles, scarlet fever, and influenza may poison certain nerves supplying the muscles of an arm or a leg, causing temporary paralysis, or even permanent laming; or they may attack the nerve of sight or of hearing and produce blindness or deafness.

A great many of the cases of paralysis and insanity are caused by alcohol. Alcohol in excess may attack the nerves supplying the arms and legs, producing severe pain and partial paralysis. It may also, after long-continued use, affect the cells of the brain itself, producing the horrible condition known as delirium tremens--a form of acute insanity with distressing delusions, in which the patient imagines that he sees rats, snakes, and other reptiles and vermin crawling over him, or in his room. Even in those who never use it to such excess as this, or indeed in those who may never become intoxicated, the long-continued use of alcohol may produce a slow poisoning and general breaking-down of the whole nervous system, causing in time the hand to tremble, the eye to become bleared and dim, the gait weak and unsteady, the memory uncertain, and the judgment poor.

Are Nervous Diseases Increasing? The direct use of the brain and nervous system has much less to do with the production of its diseases or even its serious disturbances than is usually believed. Most of these, as we have seen, are due either to the poisons of disease or alcohol, or to the fatigue-poisons, or other poisons, produced in the stomach, the liver, the muscles, or other parts of the body. The worst results of brain-work are due to the extent to which it deprives us of proper exercise and fresh air. Good, vigorous mental activity,--hard brain work, in fact,--when you are in good condition, is, if not overdone, as healthful and almost as invigorating as physical exercise or hearty play. We often hear it said that the rush and hurry of our modern strenuous life is increasing the number of mental diseases and nervous breakdowns. But there is no evidence that the strain of civilization upon our brains and nervous systems is damaging them, or that either nervous diseases or insanity are more frequent now than they used to be one hundred or five hundred years ago. In fact, all the evidence that we have points in exactly the opposite direction; for, as we have seen, most of these brain and nerve diseases are due to infectious diseases, bad food, and bad living conditions generally, all of which the progress of modern civilization is rapidly lessening and preventing.

We are collecting our insane in modern hospitals and comfortable homes, instead of letting them wander in rags about the country, and this makes them live longer and seem more numerous. But the poorest and least highly civilized classes and races have much more insanity among them than those who live under more favorable conditions.

FOOTNOTES:

[27] Some of these coal-tar remedies are Acetanilid, and Antipyrin, and Phenacetin.

CHAPTER XXII

EXERCISE AND GROWTH

Fatigue as a Danger Signal. The chief use of exercise in childhood, whether of body or mind, is to make us grow; but it can do this only by being kept within limits. Within these limits it will increase the vigor of the heart, expand the lungs, clear the brain, deepen sleep, and improve the appetite. Beyond these limits it stunts the body, dulls the brain, overstrains the heart, and spoils the appetite. How are we going to tell when these limits are being reached? Nature has provided a danger signal--fatigue, or "tiredness."

Fatigue is due, not to complete exhaustion, but to poisoning of the muscle, or nerve, by its own waste substances. If the fatigue is general, or "all over," it is from these waste substances piling up in the blood faster than the lungs, skin, and kidneys can get rid of them. In other words, fatigue is a form of self-poisoning.

We can see how it is that exercise, which, up to the point of fatigue, is both healthful and improving, when carried on after we are tired, becomes just the opposite. Fatigue is nature's signal, "Enough for this time!" That is why all methods of training for building up strength and skill, both of mind and muscle, forbid exercising beyond well-marked fatigue. If you yourself stop at this point in exercising, you will find, the next time you try that particular exercise, that you can go a little further before fatigue is felt; the third time, a little further yet; and so, by degrees, you can build up both your body and brain to the fullest development of which they are capable.

In muscular training, a series of light, quick movements, none of which are fatiguing, repeated fifteen, twenty, or a hundred times, will do much more to build up muscle and increase strength, than three or four violent, heaving strains that tax all your strength. Real athletes and skilled trainers, for instance, use half-or three-quarter-pound dumb-bells and one-or two-pound Indian clubs, instead of the five-pound dumb-bells and ten-pound clubs with which would-be athletes delight to decorate their rooms. A thoroughbred race-horse is trained on the same principle: he is never allowed to gallop until tired, or to put out his full speed before he is well grown. In fact, the best methods of all forms of exercising and training always stop just short of fatigue. Education and study ought to be planned on the same principle. Exercise of either our muscles or our minds after they have begun to poison themselves through fatigue never does them any good, even if it does not do them serious harm; and, where the exercise is for the sake of building us up and developing our powers, it is best to stop for a little while, or change the task, as soon as we begin to feel distinctly tired, and then to try it again when we are rested.

This is one of the secrets of the healthfulness and value of play and games for children, and for older persons as well. When you get tired, you can stop and rest; and then start in again when you feel rested--that is to say, when your heart has washed the poisons out of your muscles and nerves. In fact, if you will notice, you will find that nearly all play and games are arranged on this plan--a period of activity followed by a period of rest. Some games have regular "innings," with alternate activity and rest for the players; or each player takes his turn at doing the hard work; or the players are constantly changing from one thing to another--for instance, throwing or striking the ball one minute; running to first base the next; and standing on base the next. Every muscle, every sense, every part of you is exercised at once, or in rapid succession, and no part has time to become seriously fatigued; so that you can play hard all the afternoon and never once be uncomfortably tired, though your muscles have done a tremendous lot of work, measured in foot-pounds or "boy-power," in that time.

The good school imitates nature in this respect. The recitation periods are short, and recesses frequent; a heavy subject is followed by a lighter one; songs, drawing, calisthenics, and marching are mixed in with the lessons, so as to give every part of the mind and body plenty to do, and yet not over-tire any part.

All-Round Training from Work and Play. Every game that is worth playing, every kind of work that accomplishes anything worth while, trains and develops not merely the muscles and the heart, but the sight, hearing, touch, and sense of balance, and the powers of judgment, memory, and reason, as well.

If you are healthy, you know that you don't need to be told to play, or even how, or what, to play; for you would rather play than eat. You have as strong and natural an appetite for play as you have for food when you are hungry, or for water when you are thirsty, or for sleep when you are tired. It is just as right to follow the one instinct as the others, though any one may be carried to extremes.

Some of the most important part of your training and fitting for life is given by plays and games. Not only do they put you in better condition to study and enjoy your work in school, but they also teach you many valuable lessons as well. Our favorite national game, base-ball, for instance, not only develops the muscles of your arms and shoulders in throwing the ball and in striking and catching it, and your lungs and heart in rushing to catch a fly or in running the bases, but also develops quickness of sight and hearing,--requires, as we say, "a good eye" for distance,--makes you learn to calculate something of the speed at which a ball is coming toward you or flying up into the air, requires you to judge correctly how far it is to the next base and how few seconds it will take to get there and whether you or the baseman can get there first.

More important yet, like all team games, it teaches you to work with others, to obey orders promptly, to give up your own way and do, not what you like best, but what will help the team most; to keep your temper, to bend every energy to win, but to play fair. It also teaches you that you must begin at the beginning, take the lowest place, and gradually work yourself up; and that only by hard work and patience and determination can you make yourself worth anything to the team, to say nothing of becoming a "star" player.

If you will just go at your studies the way you do at base-ball, you will make a success of them. Make up your mind to gain a little at a time, to learn something new every day, and you will be astonished how your knowledge will mount up at the end of the year. When you first start in a new study, it looks, as you say, "like Greek" to you. You feel quite sure that you never will be able to understand those hard words or solve those problems "clear over in the back of the book." But remember how you started in on the diamond as a "green player," with fumbling fingers that missed half the balls thrown to you, with soft hands that stung every time you tried to stop a "hot" ball; how you ducked and flinched when a fast ball came at you, and how you fumbled half your flies and, even when you fielded them, were likely to send them in six feet over the baseman's head. But by quietly sticking to it--watching how the good players did it, and playing an hour or two every day during the season--you gradually grew into the game, until, almost without knowing how it happened, you had trained your muscles, your nerve cells, and your brain and found yourself a good batsman and a sure catcher.

So it will be in your school work. Just stick quietly to it, taking your work a lesson at a time; give yourself plenty of sleep and plenty of fresh air, and eat plenty of good food three times a day, and your mind will grow in strength and skill as gradually, as naturally, and as happily as your body does.

Every season of the year has its special games suited to the weather and the condition of the ground. If you take pride in playing all of them in their turn, hard and thoroughly, and making as good a record in them as you can, you will find that it will not only keep you healthy and make you grow, but will help you in your school work as well, by keeping your wits bright and your head clear. There is a fine group of running games, for instance, such as Prisoner's Base, or Dare Base, Hide-and-Seek, or I Spy, and the different kinds of tag,--Fox-and-Geese, Duck-on-Rock,--which are not only capital exercise for leg muscles, lungs, and heart, but fine training in quickness of sight, quickness and accuracy of judgment, and quickness of ear in catching the slightest rustle on either side, or behind you, so that you can rush back to the base, or "home," first.

Then with the winter comes skating, with hockey and Prisoner's Base on the ice, and coasting and sledding and snow-balling, to say nothing of forts and snowmen. You should try to be out of doors as many hours a day in the winter-time as in the summer, so far as possible. If you play and romp hard, you will find that you don't mind the cold at all, and that, instead of taking more colds and chills, you will have fewer of these than you had when you cooped yourself up indoors beside the warm stove.

It is just as important for girls to play all these games as it is for boys; and girls enjoy them just as much and can play them almost, if not quite, as well, if they are only allowed to begin when they are small and do just as they please. There is no reason whatever why a girl should not be just as quick of eye and ear, and as fast on the run, and as well able to throw or catch or bat a ball, as a boy. Up to fifteen years of age boys and girls alike ought to be dressed in clothes that will allow them to play easily and vigorously at any good game that happens to be in season. Girls like base-ball as well as boys do, if they are only shown how to play it.

In summer, of course, the whole wide world outdoors turns into one great playground; and it is largely because we turn out into this playground that we have so much less sickness, and so many fewer cases of the serious diseases like tuberculosis, pneumonia, and rheumatism in summer than in winter.

Boys and girls ought to know how to swim and how to handle a boat before they are twelve years old; for these are not only excellent forms of exercise and most healthful and enjoyable amusements in themselves, but they may be the means of saving lives--one's own life or the lives of others.

As a form of exercise and education combined, nothing is better than walks in the country or, where this is impossible, in parks and public gardens. An acquaintance with trees, flowers, plants, birds, and wild animals, is one of the greatest sources of enjoyment and good health that any one can have all his life through.

Last, but not by any means least, comes that delightful combination of work and play known as gardening, and the lighter forms of farming. Every child naturally delights in having a little patch of ground of his own in which he can dig and rake and weed and plant seeds and watch the plants grow. In our large cities, where most of the houses have not sufficient space about them to allow children to have gardens of their own at home, land is being bought near school-houses and laid out as school gardens, and the work done in them is counted as part of the school work. Indeed, so important is this work considered as a part of school education, that some large cities are actually building their schools out in the open country, so that they can have plenty of space for playgrounds and gardens and shops, and carrying the children from the central parts of the city out to them by trolley or train in the morning and back at night.

Wherever you happen to live, you should engage in healthy happy, vigorous play in the open air at least two to four hours a day all the year round. If you live in a town, while it will not be quite so easy to reach the woods and the fields and the swimming holes and the skating ponds, yet you will have a large number of playmates of your own age, and have good opportunity to play the games calling for half a dozen or more players; and there will be plenty of vacant lots and open spaces, or little-traveled streets, in which to play base-ball and foot-ball and Prisoner's Base and tag. And although you may not be within reach of the best zoological garden ever made,--a barnyard,--yet you can make occasional trips to the city "Zoo," or the botanical gardens, or to parks.

Healthful Methods of Study. In the growth and training of the highest, most valuable, and most wonderful part of the body--the brain--the same methods followed in our outdoor games will give the best results. We do not create intelligence by study, nor manufacture a brain for ourselves, in school. We simply develop and strengthen and improve the brains and the mental power that we were born with.

Our minds grow as our bodies do, by healthful exercise--little at a time, with plenty of rest and change of occupation between the periods of work. That is why our school studies are arranged as they are: instead of one subject being studied all the morning, or all day, four or five subjects are studied for twenty or thirty minutes each, and a change is made to another before our minds become over-tired and begin poisoning themselves with fatigue toxins. A subject that is rather hard for us is followed by one that is easier; and the hardest subjects in the course are usually taken up early in the morning session, or after recess, or early in the afternoon, when we are well-rested and feeling fresh and ready for work.

We should try to keep our bodies and our brains and our sight and hearing in the very best possible condition for our work, so as to come up to each task that we have to master keen and fresh and clear-headed, rather than to take pride in spending so many hours a day studying in a half-tired, half-hearted, listless kind of way. You will find that you will be able to master a lesson and see through a problem in half the time if you get plenty of sleep in a room with the windows open, play a great deal out-of-doors, and do not hurry through your meals for either school or play.

Study just as you play ball when you are trying to make a place on the team. Bend every energy that you have to that one thing, and forget everything else, until you have finished it. You can do more work in fifteen minutes in this way than you can in forty minutes of sitting and looking out of the window and wondering how much longer the study period is to last, and what the next chapter is about in the story that you are reading at home, or what you are going to wear to the party next week.

Keep yourself in good condition, and then buckle down to your work as if that were the only thing there was in the world for the time being, and you will be surprised to find, not only how much more easily and quickly you will do your work, but how much better you will remember it afterwards. Do not set out to accomplish too much at a time; but when you undertake a task, don't let go until you have finished it. If you will train yourself in this way, you will soon find that it will seldom take you longer to master a lesson than it will to recite it. It is becoming more and more the custom in the best schools to plan to do all the school work in school hours, alternating periods of recitation and play with periods of study, so that no school-books need be taken home at night. This cannot always be done; but it is well to come as near to it as possible, in order, first, to learn to do work quickly and thoroughly and to drop it when it is finished, and, secondly, to give time to playing and resting and forming the priceless habit of reading. You will leave school some day, but you may still be a student in the great University of Books; and the pleasure of widening your knowledge and kindling your imagination will never fail you or pall on you as long as you live. An evening spent with newspapers and magazines, with books of travel and adventure, with good stories and poetry, with enjoyable and sensible parlor games such as authors, checkers, chess, charades, and with music and singing, will help you more with your lessons next day than two hours of listless yawning over text-books.

If you take your school work in this spirit, you will find that you will enjoy it quite as well as any other form of exercise--even play itself. The harder and more intelligently you play, the better you will be able to work in the schoolroom; and the harder and more intelligently you study, the more you will enjoy your play.

CHAPTER XXIII

THE LOOKOUT DEPARTMENT

Why the Eyes, Ears, and Nose are Near the Mouth. If you had no eyes, ears, or nose, you might just as well be dead; and you soon would be, if you had no one to feed you and guide you about and take care of you. Naturally, all three of these scouts and spies of the body, which warn us of danger and guide us to food and shelter, are near the mouth, at the head-end of the body. The nose by means of which we smell food, to see whether it is sweet and good or not, is directly above the mouth; the eyes are above and on each side, like the lamps of an automobile, but swinging in sockets like search-lights; while the ears are a couple of inches behind, on each side of us, for catching from the sea of air the waves that we call sound.

You could almost guess what each of these is for, just by looking at it. The nose and the ears are open and hollow because air must pass into them in order to bring us odors or sounds; while the eyes are solid, somewhat like big glass marbles, to receive light--because light can go right through anything that is transparent. Eyes, ears, and nose all began on the surface, and sank gradually into the head, so as to be surrounded and protected, leaving just opening enough at the surface to allow smells, light-rays, and sound-waves to enter; and all of them have at their bottom, or deepest part, a sensitive patch of surface, which catches the light, or the smells, or the sounds, and sends them by a special nerve to the brain.

These three sets of organs have gradually and slowly grown into the shape in which we now find them, in order to do the particular kind of smelling, seeing, and hearing that will be most useful to us. Every kind of animal has a slightly different shape and arrangement of eye, of ear, and of nose to fit his particular "business"; but in all animals they are built upon the same simple, general plan.

THE NOSE

How the Nose is Made. The nose began as a pair of little puckers, or dimples, just above the mouth, containing cells that were particularly good smellers, in order to test the food before it was eaten. All smells rise, so these cells were right on the spot for their particular "business."

The original way of breathing, before the nose-dimples or pits opened through into the throat, was through the mouth; and that is one reason why it is so easy to fall into the bad habit of mouth-breathing whenever the nose gets blocked by adenoids or catarrh. Some creatures--fishes, for instance,-- breathe through their mouths entirely; if you watch one in an aquarium or a clear stream, you will easily see that it is going "gulp, gulp, gulp" constantly. The saying "to drink like a fish" is a slander upon an innocent creature; for what it is really doing is breathing, not drinking. Even a frog, which has nostrils opening into its throat, still has to swallow its air in gulps, as you can see by watching its throat when it is sitting quietly. And, strange as it may seem, if you prop its mouth open, it will suffocate, because it can no longer gulp down air.[28]

Our noses are nine-tenths for breathing, and only about one-tenth for smelling; so that by far the greater part of the nose is built on breathing lines. But the smelling part of it, though small, is very important, because it now has to decide, not merely upon the goodness or badness of the food, but also upon the purity or foulness of the air we breathe. The nostrils lie, as you can see, side by side, separated from each other by a thin, straight plate of gristle and bone known as the septum. This should be perfectly straight and flat; but very often when the nose does not grow properly in childhood, it becomes crumpled upon itself, or bulged over to one side or the other, and so blocks up one of the nostrils. This is a very common cause of catarrh, and requires, for its cure, a slight operation, a cutting away of the bulging or projecting part of the septum. The rims of the openings of the nose, known as the wings, have little muscles fastened to them which pull them upward and backward, thus widening the air openings or, as we say, dilating the nostrils. If you will watch any one who has been running fast, or a horse that has been galloping, you will see that his nostrils enlarge with every breath; and these same movements occur in sick people who are suffering from disease of the lungs or the heart, which makes it difficult for them to get breath enough.

Each nostril opens into a short and rather narrow, but high, passage, known as the nasal passage, through which the air pours into the back of the throat, or pharynx, and so down into the windpipe and lungs. Instead of having smooth walls, however, the passage is divided into three almost separate tubes, by little shelves of bone that stick out from the outer wall. These are covered with thick coils of tiny blood vessels, through which hot blood is being constantly pumped, like steam through the coils of a radiator, so that the air, as it is being drawn into the lungs, is warmed and moistened. The passage is lined with a soft, moist "skin," called mucous membrane, very much like that which lines the stomach and bowels, except that it is covered with tiny little microscopic hairs, called cilia, and that its glands pour out a thin, sticky mucus, instead of a digestive juice. This thick network of blood vessels just under the thin mucous "skin" is easily scratched into or broken, and then we have "nose-bleed."

The purpose of this mucus is to catch and hold, just as flypaper catches flies, all specks of dust, lint, or germs that may be floating in the air we breathe, and to keep them from going on into the lungs. As these are caught upon the lining of the nose, they are washed down by the flow of mucus or wafted by the movement of the tiny hairs back into the throat, and swallowed into the stomach, where they are digested. Or, if they are very irritating, they are blown out of the nostrils, or sneezed out, and in that way got rid of.

If the dust is too irritating, or the air is foul and contains disease germs, these set up an inflammation in the nose, and we "catch cold," as we say. If we keep on breathing bad or dusty air, the walls of the nasal passages become permanently thickened and swollen; the mucus, instead of being thin and clear, becomes thick and sticky and yellowish, and we have a catarrh.

Catarrh is the result of a succession of neglected "bad colds," caused, not by fresh, cold air, but by hot, stuffy, foul air containing dust and germs. The best and only sure way to avoid catarrh is by breathing nothing but fresh, pure air, day and night, keeping your skin clean and vigorous by cool bathing every day, and taking plenty of play in the open air.

So perfect is this heating, warming, and dust-cleansing apparatus in the nose, that by the time quite cold air has passed through the nostrils, and got down into the back of the throat, it has been warmed almost to the temperature of the body, or blood-heat, and has been moistened and purified of three-fourths of its dust or disease germs. When you go out of doors on a cold, frosty morning, your nose is very likely to block up, because so much hot blood is pumped into these little steam-coils of blood vessels, in order to warm the air properly, that they swell until they almost block up the nostrils.

The Sense of Smell. The lower three-fourths of the nasal passages have nothing whatever to do with the sense of smell; this is found only in the highest, or third, division of the passages, right up under the root of the nose, where odors can readily rise to it. Here can be found a little patch of mucous membrane of a deep yellowish color, which is very sensitive to smells, and from which a number of tiny little nerve twigs run up to form the nerve of smell (olfactory nerve), which goes directly to the brain. The position of the smell area at the highest and narrowest part of the nose passage explains why when you have a very bad cold, you almost lose your sense of smell; the lining of the lower part of the nose has become so inflamed and swollen as to block up the way to the highest part where the smelling is done.

Adenoids. If colds are neglected and allowed to run on, the inflammation spreads through the nose back into the upper part of the throat, or pharynx. Here it attacks a spongy group of glands, like a third tonsil, which swells up until it almost blocks up the nose and makes you breathe through your mouth. These swollen glands are called adenoids, and cause not only mouth-breathing, but deafness, loss of appetite, indigestion, headache, and a stupid, tired condition; so that children that are mouth-breathers are often two or more grades behind in school, poor students, and even stunted and undersized. You can often tell them at sight by their open mouths and vacant, stupid look. A very simple and harmless scraping operation will remove these adenoids entirely, and what a wonderful improvement the mouth-breather will make! He will often catch up two grades, and gain two inches in height and ten pounds in weight within a year.

Adenoids not only cause deafness by blocking up the tube (Eustachian) that runs from the throat to the ear,--the tube through which the air passes when your ear "goes pop,"--but are also the commonest cause of ear-ache and gatherings in the ear, which may burst the drum.

THE TONGUE

The Tongue is not Used chiefly for Tasting. If you will notice the next time that you have a bad cold, you will find that you have almost lost your sense of taste, as well as of smell, so that everything tastes "flat" to you. This illustrates what scientists have known for a long time, but which seems very hard to believe, that two-thirds of what we call taste is really smell. If you carefully block up your nostrils with cotton or wax, so that no air can possibly reach the smell region at the top of them, and blindfold your eyes, and have some one cut a raw potato, an apple, and a raw onion into little pieces of the same size and shape, and put them into your mouth one after the other, you will find that it is difficult to tell which is which.

The only tastes that are really perceived in the mouth are bitter, sweet, sour, and salty; and even these are perceived quite as much by the roof and back of the mouth, especially the soft palate, as they are by the tongue. All the delicate flavors of our food, such as those of coffee or of roast meat or of freshly baked bread, are really smells.

The tongue, which is usually described as the organ of taste, is really a sort of fingerless hand grown up from the floor of the mouth--to help suck in or lap up water or milk, push the food in between the teeth for chewing, and, when it has been chewed, roll it into a ball and push it backward down the throat. It is not even the chief organ of speech; for people who have had their tongues removed on account of cancer, or some other disease, can talk fairly well, although not so clearly as with the whole tongue.

The tongue is simply a "tongue-shaped" bundle of muscles, covered with a thick, tough skin of mucous membrane, dotted all over with little knob-like processes called papill? which are of various shapes, but of no particular utility, except to roughen the surface of the tongue and give it a good grip on the food. If the mucous "skin" covering the tongue does not shed off properly, the dead cells on its surface become thickened and whitish, and the germs of the mouth begin to breed and grow in them, forming a sort of mat over the surface. Then we say that the tongue is badly coated. This coating is in part due to unhealthy conditions of the stomach and bowels, and in part to lack of proper cleaning of the mouth and teeth.

The Sense of Taste can usually be Trusted. Since the nose and the tongue have had about five million years' experience in picking out what is good and refusing what is bad, their judgment is pretty reliable, and their opinion entitled to the greatest respect. As a general thing, those things that taste good are wholesome and nutritious; the finest and most enjoyable flavors known are those of our commonest and most wholesome foods, such as good bread, fresh butter, roast meats, apples, cheese, sugar, fruit, etc.; while, on the other hand, those things that taste bad or bitter or salty or sour, or that we have to learn to like, like beer or pickles or strong cheese or tea or coffee, are more often unwholesome or have little nutritive value. Very few real foods taste bad when we first try them. If we used our noses to test every piece of food that went into our mouths, and refused to eat it if it "smelt bad," we should avoid many an attack of indigestion and ptomaine poisoning. It is really a great pity that it is not considered polite to "sniff" at the table.

THE EYE

How the Eye is Made. Next in importance after the smell and the taste of our food comes the appearance of it; hence, our need of eyes to help us in choosing what to eat, as well as how to avoid the dangers about us.

The eyes began as little sensitive spots on the surface of the head. Like the nose pits, as they became more sensitive, they too sank in beneath the surface; but with this difference, that, instead of remaining open, the rims or edges of the eye-pit grew together and became transparent, forming a cover, or eye-glass, which became the clear part of the eye, called the cornea. At the same time, the little sensitive spot at the bottom of the eye-pit spread out into the shape of the bottom of a cup, called the retina; and then the hollow of that cup between the retina and the cornea filled up with a clear, soft, animal jelly called the vitreous humor, and we have the eye as it is in our heads to-day.

The sensitive retina, spreading out, as it does, to form the back of the eyeball, is the nerve-coat of the eye; and from its centre a thick round bundle of nerve fibres, known as the optic nerve, runs back to the brain.

The bones of the head, grown out in a ring in order to protect the eyes, are called the orbit or socket.

To protect the delicate glass (cornea) of the eye, there are two folds of skin, one above and one below, known as the eyelids. The eyelids carry a row of extra long hairs at their edges, called the eyelashes, and a number of little glands, somewhat like those of the stomach, to pour out a fluid, which makes the lids glide smoothly over the eyeball and keeps them from sticking together. Underneath the upper lid a number of these glands become gathered together and "grow in," after the fashion of the salivary glands, to form a larger gland about the size of a small almond, which pours out large amounts of this fluid as tears. It is called the tear gland (lachrymal gland).

Whenever a cinder or a grain of sand or a tiny insect or any other irritating thing gets into the eye, this gland pours out a flood of tears, which washes the intruder down into the inner corner of the eye where it can be wiped out; or, if it be small enough, carries it down through a little tube in the edge of each eyelid, through a little passage known as the nasal, or tear, duct, into the nose. So, if you get anything into your eye, much the best and safest thing to do is to hold the lids half shut, but as loose, or relaxed, as possible, and allow the tears to wash the speck of dust down into the inner corner of the eye. If you squeeze down too hard with the lids, and particularly if you rub the eye, you will be very likely to scratch the cornea with the speck of dust or sand, or, if the speck be sharp-edged, to drive it right into the cornea and give yourself a great deal of unnecessary pain and trouble, or even seriously damage the eye. If the cinder or dust doesn't wash down quickly, pull the upper lid gently away from the eyeball by the lashes and hold it there a minute or so, when often the cinder will drop or wash out.

As the light rays cannot be bent, or drawn into the eyes as smells can into the nostrils, it is necessary that the eyes should be able to roll about so as to turn in different directions; and so nature has made them round, or globular, attaching to their outer coat or shell (the sclerotic coat) little bands of muscle, each of which pulls the eyeball in its particular direction. There are four straight bands--one for each point of the compass: one fastened to the upper surface of the eye to roll it upward; another to the lower to roll it downward; another to the outer to roll it outward; and another to the inner side to roll it inward for near vision.[29]

There is another reason for the rounded shape of the eye--that it may act as a lens in condensing the rays of light. In order that we may see things clearly, the rays of light must be brought to a focus upon or close to the retina, at the back of the eye; and our eyes are so shaped that they form a lens of proper thickness, or strength, to do this.

You can see how this is done with an ordinary magnifying glass, or burning-glass. The little sharply lighted and heated point to which the light-rays can be brought is the focus of the lens, and the distance it lies behind the lens is called the focal distance. The thicker the lens, or burning-glass, is in the middle, the shorter its focal distance, and the more strongly it will magnify.

A healthy, or normal, eye is of just such shape and "bulge" that rays of light entering the eye are brought to a focus on, or close to, the retina at the back of the eyeball. Some people, however, are unfortunately born with eyes that are too small and flat, or do not "bulge" enough; and then the rays of light are focused behind the retina instead of upon it, and the image is blurred. This is known as "long sight" (hyperopia), and can be corrected by putting in front of the eyes lenses of glass, called spectacles, which bulge sufficiently to bring the rays to focus on the retina.

An eye that is too large and round and bulging brings the rays to a focus in front of the retina, and this also blurs the image. This form of poor sight is called "short sight" (myopia), and can be relieved by putting in front of the eye a glass that is concave, or thinnest in the middle and thickest at the edges, in the right proportions to focus the image where it belongs, right on the retina. This kind of glass is sometimes called a "minifying" glass, from the fact that it makes objects seen through it look smaller. It is also called a "minus" glass, while the magnifying glass is called a "plus" glass. The shape of the glasses or spectacles prescribed for an eye is just the opposite of that of the eye. If the eye is too flat (long-sighted), you put on a bulging, or convex, glass;

and if the eye is too bulging (short-sighted), a hollow, or concave, glass. Other eyes are irregularly shaped in front and bulge more in one direction than another, like an orange. This defect is called astigmatism and is very troublesome, making it hard to fit the eye with glasses, as the glasses have to be ground irregular in shape.

We have just seen how the eye deals with rays of light coming from a distance, which are practically parallel. When, however, books or other objects are brought near the eye, the rays of light coming from them do not remain parallel, but begin to spread apart, or diverge; and a stronger lens is required to bring them to a focus upon the retina. To provide for this, there is in the middle of the eyeball a firm, elastic, little globular body about the size and shape of a lemon-drop, called the crystalline lens. Around this is a ring of muscle, which is so arranged that when it contracts it causes the lens to change its shape and become more bulging, or thicker in the middle. This makes the eyeball a "stronger" lens so that the rays of light can be brought to a focus upon the retina.

This action is known as accommodation, or adjustment; and you can sometimes feel it going on in your own eye, as when you pick up a book or a piece of sewing and bring it up quickly, close to the eye, in order to see clearly.

If this little muscle is worked too hard, as when we try to read in a bad light, it becomes tired and we get what is called "eye-strain"; and if the strain be kept up too long, it will give us headache and may even make us sick at the stomach. The commonest cases of eye-strain are in eyes that are too flat (hyperopic) where this little muscle has to "bulge" the lens enough to make good the defect and bring the rays to a focus. This, however, of course keeps it on a constant strain; and the eye is continually giving out, and its owner suffering from headache, neuralgia, dyspepsia, sleeplessness, and other forms of nervous trouble, until the proper lens or spectacle is fitted.[30]

A surface as delicate and sensitive to light as the retina, would, of course, be damaged by too bright a glare; so in the front of the eye, just behind the cornea, a curtain has grown up, with an opening or "peep-hole" in its centre, which can be enlarged or made smaller by little muscles. This opening is the pupil; the curtain, which is colored so as to shut out the rays of light, is known as the iris, for the quaint, but rather picturesque, reason that Iris in Greek means "rainbow," and this part of the eye may be any one of its colors.

The Care of the Eyes. The most dangerous diseases of the eye are caused by infectious germs, which get into them either from the outside, as in dust, or by touching them with dirty fingers; or through the blood, as in measles, smallpox, tuberculosis, and rheumatism. The more completely we can prevent these diseases, the less blindness we shall have in the nation. About one-sixth of all cases of blindness in our asylums is caused by a germ that gets into babies' eyes at birth, but can be done away with by proper washing and cleansing of the eyes.

THE EAR

Structure of the Ear. Next after sight, hearing is our most important sense; without it, speaking, and consequently reading and writing, would be impossible. Man learned to speak by hearing the sounds made by other people and things, and then by listening to his own voice and practicing until he could imitate them. Children who are unfortunate enough to be born deaf also become dumb, not because there is anything the matter with their voice organs, but simply because, as they cannot hear the sounds they make, they do not form them by practice into words and sentences. By proper training, deaf mutes can now be taught to speak, though their voices sound flat and "tinny," like a phonograph.

As in the nose and the eye, the important part of the ear is the nerve spot that can "feel" the air waves that we call sound, just as the retina "feels" light. It is from this sensitive spot that the auditory nerve carries the sound to the brain. This spot has grown into quite an elaborate structure, buried, for safety, deeply in the bones of the skull, close to the base of the brain. It is made up of a long row of tiny little nerve rods, laid side by side like the keys of a piano, only there are about three thousand of them. Each one of these is supposed to respond, or vibrate, to a particular tone, or sound. This keyboard, from the fact that, to save space, it is coiled upon itself like a sea-shell, instead of running straight, is called the cochlea (Greek for "snail-shell"); it is also called, because it is the deepest, or innermost, part of the hearing apparatus, the internal ear.

Just as the retina has a lens and a vitreous humor in front of it to act upon the light, so the internal ear has an apparatus in front of it to act upon the sound waves. This is called the drum (tympanum). It consists of a fold of thin, delicate skin stretched tightly across the bottom of the outer ear canal, as parchment is stretched across the head of a drum. If you should take a hand-mirror--best a hollow, or concave, one--and throw a bright ray of light deep into some one's ear, you would be able, after a little trying, to see this drum-skin stretched across the bottom of it and about an inch and a quarter in from the surface of the head.

When the sound waves go into the ear canal and strike upon this tiny drum, which is about two-thirds the size of a silver dime and really more like a tambourine or the disk of a telephone or phonograph than a drum, they start it thrilling, or vibrating, just as a guitar string vibrates when you thrum it. These little vibrations are carried across the hollow behind the drum by a chain of tiny bones, known as the ear-bones (called from their shapes, the hammer, the anvil, and the stirrup), and passed on to the keyboard of the cochlea.

Here comes in one of the most curious things about this ingenious hearing-apparatus. This little hollow behind the drum-skin has to be kept full of air in order to let the drum vibrate properly, and this is arranged for by a little tube (the Eustachian tube) which runs down from the bottom of it and opens into the back of the throat just behind the nasal passages, and above the soft palate. When you blow your nose very hard, you will sometimes feel one of your ears go "pop"; and that means that you have blown a bubble of air out through this tube into your drum cavity.

If your nose and throat become inflamed, then the mouth of this little tube may become blocked up; the drum can no longer thrill, or vibrate, properly; and, for the time being, you are deaf. This tube is of great importance, because nearly all the diseases that attack the ear start in at the throat and travel up the tube until they reach the drum cavity. This is why one so often has earache after an attack of the grip or after a bad cold. The drum cavity, with its chain of bones and its tube down to the throat, is called, from its position, the middle ear.

The outer, or external, ear, though far the largest of the three parts, and quite imposing in appearance, is really of little use or importance. It is simply a sort of receiving trumpet for catching sounds, with a very wide and curiously curved and crumpled mouth, or bell. The large, expanded mouth of the trumpet, called the concha ("conch shell"), was at one time capable of being "pricked up" and turned in the direction of sounds, just as horses' or dogs' ears are now; and in our own ears there are still for this purpose three pairs of tiny unused muscles running from them to the side of the head. But the concha is now motionless and almost useless, except for its beauty; and it is very troublesome to wash.

The Care of the Ear. The tube of the trumpet leading down from the surface of the ear to the drum is lined with skin; and this skin is supplied with glands, which pour out a sticky, yellowish fluid called ear wax, which catches the bits of dust or insects that get into the ear and, flowing slowly outward, carries them with it. If it is let alone, it will keep the ear canal clean and healthy; but some people imagine that, because it looks yellowish, it must be dirt; and consequently, from mistaken ideas of cleanliness, they work at it with the end of the finger, the corner of a towel, or even with a hairpin, an ear-spoon, or an ear-pick, and in this way stop the proper flow of the wax and make it dry and block up the ear.

Remember, you should not wash too deeply into your ears; (as the old German proverb puts it, "Never pick your ear with anything smaller than your elbow"). And if you don't, you will seldom have trouble with wax in the ear. Scarcely one case of deafness in a hundred is caused by wax. When your ear does become blocked up with wax, it is best to go to a doctor and let him syringe it out. Picking at it, or even syringing too hard, may do serious damage to the ear.

If an earache is neglected, the inflammation may spread into some air-cells in the bony lump behind the ear (the mastoid) and thus cause mastoid disease, which may spread to, and attack, the brain if not cured by a surgical operation.

OUR SPIRIT-LEVELS

The Sixth Sense. Though we usually speak of having five senses,--sight, smell, hearing, touch, and taste,--we really have also a sixth--the sense of direction, or of balance. The "machine" of this sense is comparatively simple, being made up of three tiny curved tubes, which, from their shape, are called the semi-circular canals. These are buried in the same bone of the skull as the internal ear, and so close to it that they were at one time described as part of it. These little canals are three in number, one for each of the dimensions-- length, breadth, and thickness,--so that whichever way the head or body is moved,--backward and forward, up and down, or from side to side,--the fluid with which they are filled will change its level in one of them, just as the "bead" does in the carpenter's spirit-level that you can find in any tool shop. The delicate nerve twigs that run out into the fluid in these tiny canals are gathered together into a bundle, or nerve-cable, which runs back to the part of the brain known as the cerebellum or hind-brain, which has most to do with controlling the balance and movements of our bodies.

It is the disturbance set up in these spirit-level canals by the pitching and rolling of a ship, which makes us seasick. Neither the stomach, nor anything that we may have eaten, has anything to do with it. In the same way we sometimes become sick and dizzy from swinging too long or too high, or from riding on the cars.

FOOTNOTES:

[28] To show in how many different ways nature may carry out the same purpose, the smelling organs in insects, lobsters, and crabs are on the ends and sides of tiny feelers, which they wave about; and the eyes in lobsters, crawfish, and snails, are on the ends of stalks, which they thrust about in all directions as a burglar handles a bull's-eye lantern. Snakes "hear," or catch the sound-waves, with their flickering, forked tongues; and grasshoppers and locusts have "ear-drums" on the sides of their chests.

[29] These are called the recti or "straight" muscles, upper, lower, inner, and outer, according to their position. Then, to roll the eye round and round, there are two little muscles, one above and one below, which run "crosswise" of the orbit, called the upper and lower oblique muscles.

[30] The retina is chiefly made up of a great number of fine little nerve cells called, from their shape, the rods and cones. These are kept soaked in a colored fluid called the retinal purple, which changes under the influence of

light, somewhat in the same way that the film on a photographic plate does, thus forming pictures, which are translated by the rods and cones and telegraphed along the fibres of the optic nerve to the brain. Naturally, all parts of the retina are not equally sensitive to light; its centre, which is directly opposite the pupil of the eye, is far the most so, while those around the rim of the cup are dull. This is why, when you are looking, say at some one's face across the room, only the face and a few inches around it are seen perfectly clear and sharp, while the rest of the room is seen only vaguely.

[31] As the inside of the eye is dark, or comparatively so, the pupil, or little opening in the centre of the iris, looks black, and was at one time supposed to be a solid body instead of a hole. You can easily watch the pupil changing in size, according to the brightness of the light, from a mere pin-point in very bright sunlight or gaslight, up to the size of the butt-end of a lead pencil in the dark or in a dim light.

This change in size is very simply but ingeniously carried out by two sets of tiny muscles. One set of these muscles runs in a ring right around the pupil; and when they shorten, the opening is contracted or narrowed. The other set runs outward through the iris like the spokes of a wheel; and when they shorten, they pull the pupil open. If anyone has had "drops" (atropin) put into his eyes in order to have them fitted with glasses, he will know what a disagreeably dazzling thing it is to have the pupil permanently enlarged, so that it cannot contract in a bright light.

CHAPTER XXIV

THE SPEECH ORGANS

The Voice, a Waste Product. It is one of the most curious things in this body of ours that what we regard as its most wonderful power and gift, the voice, is, in one sense, a waste product. So ingenious is nature that she has actually made that marvelous musical instrument--the human voice--with its range, its flexibility, and its powers of expression, out of spent breath, or used-up air, which has done its work in the lungs and is being driven off to get rid of it. It is like using the waste from a kitchen sink to turn a mill.

The organs that make the human voice were never built for that purpose in the first place. Unlike the eye and the ear, nature built no special organ for the voice alone, but simply utilized the windpipe and lung-bellows, the swallowing parts of the food passage (tongue, lips, and palate) and the nose, for that purpose, long after they had taken their own particular shapes for their own special ends.

The important point about this is that a good voice requires not merely a large and well-developed "music box" in the windpipe, but good lungs, a well-shaped healthy throat, properly arched jaws,--which mean good, sound teeth,--clear and healthy nasal passages, and a flexible elastic tongue. Of course, the blood and the nerves supplying all these structures must be in good condition, as well. So practically, a good voice requires that the whole body should be healthy; and whatever we do to improve the condition of our nose, our teeth, our throat, our lungs, our digestion, and our circulation will help to improve the possibilities of our voice. There are, of course, many exceptions; but you will generally find that great singers have not only splendid lungs and large vocal cords, but good hearts, vigorous constitutions, and bodies above the average in both stature and strength.

How the Voice is Produced. The chief parts of the breathing machine that nature has made over for talking purposes are the windpipe, or air tube, and the muscles in its walls. In the neck, about three inches above the collar bone, four or five of the rings of cartilage, or gristle,--which, you remember, give stiffening to the windpipe,--have grown together and enlarged to form a voice box, or larynx.

The upper edge of this voice box forms the projection in the front of the throat known by the rather absurd name of the "Adam's apple." This grows larger in proportion to the heaviness of the sounds to be made, and hence is larger in men than in women and boys. When the boy's voice box begins to grow to the man's in shape and size, his voice is likely to "break"; for it is changing from the high, clear boy's voice to the heavy, deep voice of the man.

Inside of this voice box, one of the rings of muscle that run around the windpipe has stretched into a pair of straight, elastic bands, or strings, one on each side of the air pipe, known as the vocal cords, or voice bands. These are so arranged that they can be stretched and relaxed by little muscles; and, when thrown into vibration by the air rushing through the voice box, they produce the sounds that we call talking or singing. The more tightly they are stretched, the higher and shriller are the tones they produce; and the more they are slackened, or relaxed, the deeper and more rumbling are the tones.

This is why, when you try to sing a high note, you can feel something tightening and straining in your throat, until finally you can stretch it no tighter, and your voice "breaks," as you say, into a scream or cry.

All musical instruments that have strings, are played, or produce their sounds, upon this same principle. The thinner and shorter the string, or the more tightly it is stretched, the higher the note; the heavier and longer the string, the lower the note. But no musical instrument ever yet invented can equal the human voice in the music of its tones, in its range, in the different variety and quality of tones it can produce, and in its wonderful power of expression. The human voice is a combination of reed organ, pipe organ, trumpet, and violin; and can produce in its tiny music box--only about two inches long by one inch wide--all the tones and qualities of tones that can be produced on all these instruments, except that it cannot go quite so high or so low.

All the musical instruments in the world, from the penny whistle to the grand piano, are but poor imitations of the human music box. The bellows, of course, of the human pipe organ are the lungs; while the tongue furnishes the stops; and the throat, mouth, and nose, the resonance, or sounding, chambers.

Just as a violin, or guitar, has two main parts,--a string, which vibrates and makes the sound; and a box, or hollow body, which catches that sound and enlarges it and gives it sweetness and vibration and quality,--so the human voice has two similar parts--the vocal bands, which make the sound; and a sound box, or rather series of three resonance boxes,--the throat, the mouth, and the nasal passages,--which enlarge and soften it and improve its quality.

You would naturally think that the strings, or cords, were the most important part both of the voice and of a musical instrument; and in one sense they are, as it could make no noise at all without them. But in another sense, far more important are the sounding boxes, or resonance chambers. The whole quality and value, for instance, of a Stradivarius[32] violin, which will make it readily bring ten thousand dollars in the open market, are due to the skill with which the body, or sound box, was made; the quality of the wood used; and, odd as it may seem, even the varnish used on it--the strings are the same as on any five-dollar fiddle. This is almost equally true of the human voice. While its size, or volume, is determined by the voice box and vocal bands, and its power largely by the lungs and chest, its musical quality, its color, and its expression are given almost entirely by the throat, mouth (including the lips), and nose. The proper management of these parts is two-thirds of voice training, and all these are largely under our control.

How a Good Voice may be Developed. If the nasal passages, for instance, are blocked by a bad cold or a catarrh or adenoids, then nearly half the body of your violin is blocked up and deadened; half your resonance chamber is destroyed, and the voice sounds flat and dead and nasal. If, on the other hand, your throat be swollen, or blocked, as by enlarged tonsils or chronic sore throat, then this part of the resonance chamber is muffled and spoiled, and your voice will be either entirely gone or hoarse; though perhaps by driving it very hard you may be able to make a clear tone.

If you have an attack of inflammation or cold further down, and the vocal bands swell, or the mucous membrane lining the voice box becomes inflamed and thickened, then the voice is lost entirely, just as the tone of a violin would be if a wet cloth were thrown across the strings. But disturbances in the voice box, or larynx, cause only a very small percentage of husky, poor, or unmusical voices.

A far commoner cause, indeed probably the commonest single cause of a poor, squeaky, or drawling, unmusical voice is careless and improper management of the mouth and lips. In the first place, you can easily show that such marked differences in sound as those of the different vowels are all produced by the mouth and lips. If you will prepare to say the vowels--a, e, i, o, u--aloud, and begin with a, and then hold your mouth and lips firmly in the same position, you will find that all the other vowels also come out as a. If, on the other hand, you begin with your mouth and lips in the rounded and somewhat thrust-out position necessary to say o, and try to repeat the rest of the vowels, you will find that you cannot say them at all, but only different forms of o. When you have convinced yourself of this, repeat the vowels loudly and clearly without stopping to think about the position of the mouth, and notice how your lips, the tip and base of your tongue, and your soft palate and throat all change their positions for each successive vowel.

If you will try to sing the scale, beginning with a comfortable note about the middle of your voice range, and letting your mouth take the shape for that note unconsciously, you will find that, as you sing up the scale, you change the shape of your mouth, lips, and tongue at every note, thrusting the lips and mouth further forward as if to whistle, narrowing the opening and closing up the back of your throat for the high notes.

On the other hand, as you sing down, you tend to open the mouth and lips more widely, to drop the bottom of your mouth--that is, the base of your tongue--toward your throat, and your chin down toward your chest. Again you will find, just as in the case of the different vowels, that you can sing any tone clearly and musically after putting the mouth in precisely the shape that best fits that tone; and learning how to do this is a most important part of vocal training.

What we call words are simply breath sounds and voice-box sounds chopped into convenient lengths by the movements of the tongue and lips and throat. So when we come to the question of clear and pleasant speaking, or, as we term it, articulation, the lips and tongue have almost everything to do with making the difference between a clear, musical, and refined enunciation, which is so easy to understand that it is a pleasure to listen to it, and a slurred, drawling, squeaky, nasal kind of speech, which is as hard to understand as it is unpleasant to listen to.

Few of us can ever hope to develop a really great singing voice; but anyone who will take the pains can acquire a clear, distinct, and pleasing speaking voice; and perhaps half of us can learn to sing fairly well. But to do this, we must first have good, healthy, well-developed lungs and elastic chest walls, which can come only from plenty of vigorous exercise in the open air, combined with good food and well-ventilated rooms. We must have a healthy stomach, which will not fill up with gas and keep our diaphragms from going down and enlarging our chests properly; we must have clear nasal passages, good teeth, well-shaped mouths and flexible lips, which we are willing to use vigorously in articulating, or cutting up our voice sounds; and we must have good hearing and a well-trained ear. In short, the best way to get a clear, strong, pleasant voice is to have a vigorous, well-grown, healthy body.

FOOTNOTES:

[32] A famous violin-maker who lived about 200 years ago in Cremona, Italy. Fifty thousand dollars has been asked for an unusually choice "Strad."

CHAPTER XXV

THE TEETH, THE IVORY KEEPERS OF THE GATE

Why the Teeth are Important. The teeth are a very important part of our body and deserve far more attention and better care than they usually get. They are the first and most active part of our digestive system, cutting up and grinding foods that the stomach would be unable to melt without their help. In all animals except those that have horns or fists, the teeth are their most important weapons of attack and defense. So important are they in all animals, including ourselves, and so closely do they fit their different methods of food-getting and of attack and defense, that when scientists wish to decide what class, or group, a particular animal belongs to, they look first and longest at its teeth.

The shape and position of the teeth literally make the lower half of the face and give it half its expression. A properly grown and developed set of teeth not only is necessary to health and comfort, but helps greatly to make the face and expression attractive or unattractive. Few faces with bright eyes, clear skin, and white, regular, well-kept teeth are unpleasing to look at. Beauty and health are closely related, and we ought to try to have both. In fact, nine times out of ten, what we call beauty is the outward and visible sign of inward health. The healthier you are, the handsomer you'll be.

It is particularly important to understand the natural growth and proper care of the teeth because there are few organs in the body for which we are able to do so much by direct personal attention. Our stomachs, our livers, and our kidneys, for instance, are entirely out of sight, and more or less out of reach; but our teeth are both easily got at and in full view; and, to a large degree, upon the care that we give them while they are young, will depend not only their regularity and whiteness, but also the length of their life and the vigor and comfort of our digestion all our lives.

The first thing to be remembered about the teeth is that, hard and shiny and different from almost everything else in the body as they look, they are simply a part of the skin lining the mouth, hardened and shaped for their special work of biting and chewing. Much of the care needed to prevent decay should be given, not to the teeth themselves directly, but to the gums and the mucous membrane of the whole mouth. The gums and the mouth literally grew the teeth in the first place; and when they become diseased, they secrete acids which slowly eat away the crowns and roots of the teeth. Their diseases come chiefly from irritation by decaying scraps of food, or from the blocking of the nose so that air is breathed in through the mouth, drying and cracking the soft mucous membrane. After the acids from the diseased gums have attacked the teeth, the poisons of the germs that breed in the warmth and moisture of the mouth cause the teeth to decay. Eight times out of ten, if you take care of the gums the teeth will take care of themselves.

Structure of the Teeth. The upper half of the tooth, which pushes through and stands up above the jaw and the gum, we call the crown; and this is the portion that is covered with enamel, or "living glass." The body of the tooth under the enamel is formed of a hard kind of bone called dentine. The lower half of the tooth, which still is buried in the jaw, we call the root. Wrenching the lower or root part of the tooth loose from its socket in the jaw is what hurts so when a tooth is pulled. The crown of the tooth is hollow, and this hollow is filled with a soft, sensitive pulp, in which we feel toothache. Tiny blood vessels and nerve-twigs run up from the jaw to supply this pulp through canals in the roots of the tooth.

Kinds of Teeth. If you look at your own teeth in a mirror, the first thing that strikes you is your broad, white, shiny front teeth, four above and four below, shaped like the blade of a rather blunt chisel. Their shape tells what they are used for. Like chisels, they cut, or bite, the food into appropriate sizes and lengths for chewing between the back teeth; and from this use they are called the incisors, or "cutters." From having been used for so many generations upon the kind of food we live on, they have grown broader than the canines, the teeth next to them, and almost as long.

The canines are of a cone-like shape, although it is a pretty blunt cone, or peg. Those in the upper jaw lie almost directly under the centre of each eye, and are called the "eye-teeth"; though their proper name, from the fact that they are the most prominent teeth in the dog, is the canine teeth. These are our oldest and least changed teeth; and as you might guess from their shape, like a heavy, blunt spear-head, were originally the fighting and tearing teeth, and still have the longest and heaviest roots of any teeth in our jaws. If you slip your finger up under your upper lip, you can feel the great ridge of this root, standing out from the surface of the gum.

Lastly, looking farther back into our mouths, we see behind our canines a long row of broad, flat-topped, square-looking teeth, which fill up the largest part of our jaws. Again their shape tells what they are used for. They are not sharp enough to cut with, or pointed enough to tear with, but are just suited for crushing and grinding into a pulp, between their broad, flat tops, any food that may be placed between them; and from this grinding they are called the molars, or "mill" teeth. If you will look closely at the back ones, you will see that each of them has four corners, or cusps, with a cross-shaped, sunken furrow in the centre, where they come together. After they have been used in grinding food for some years and rubbing against each other, these little corner projections become worn away, and their tops become almost flat. Those in the upper jaw have three roots, and those in the lower jaw have two, so that they are solidly anchored for their heavy, grinding work. The first two molars in each jaw, behind the canines, are smaller than the others and made up of only two pieces instead of four, and hence are called the bicuspids, or "two-cusped" teeth.

As we are what the scientists call an omnivorous, or "all-devouring," animal, able to eat and live upon practically every kind of food that any animal on earth can deal with,--animal and vegetable, soft and hard, wet and dry; fruits, nuts, crabs, roots, seaweeds, insects, anything that we can get our teeth into,--we have kept in working condition some of every kind of teeth possessed by any living animal; and the most important rule for keeping our teeth in health is to give all these kinds something to do.

Just as in other animals the teeth appear when needed, and grow into the shape required, so they grow in our own mouths when they are wanted, and of the size and shape required at the time. We are born without any teeth at all; and it is only when we begin to need a little solid food added to our milk diet,--when we are about seven months old,--that our first teeth appear; and these are incisors, first of all in the lower jaw. Then, at average intervals of about three months, the other incisors and the canines appear and, last of all, the molars, so that at about two years of age we have a complete set of twenty teeth. These are called the milk teeth.

Most animals (mammals) have formed the habit of growing two sets of teeth--a smaller, slighter set for use during the first few months or years of life, and a larger, heavier set to come in and take their place after the jaws have grown to somewhat more nearly their permanent size. In our mouths, at about seven years of age, a larger, heavier tooth pushes up behind the last milk tooth,--called the "seventh year molar,"--the milk teeth begin to loosen and fall out, and their places are taken by other new teeth budding up out of the jaw just as the first set did. These take a still longer time to grow, so that the last four of the full set of thirty-two do not come through the gums until somewhere between our eighteenth and twentieth years. These last four teeth, for the rather absurd reason that they do not appear until we are old enough to be wise, are known as the "wisdom teeth." Instead of being, as one might expect, the hardest and longest-lived of all our teeth, they are the smallest and worst built of our molars and among the first of our permanent teeth to break down and disappear. Not only so, but our jaws are so much shorter than they were in the days when man fought with his teeth and knew nothing about cooking and had no tools or utensils with which to grind and prepare his food, that there is scarcely room in them for these last teeth to come through. They often cause a great deal of pain in the process, and may even break through at the side of the jaw and cause abscesses and other troubles.

Care of the Teeth. The most important thing for the health of any organ in the body is to give it plenty of exercise, and this is especially true of our teeth. This exercise can be secured by thoroughly chewing, or masticating, all our food, of whatever sort, especially breads, biscuits, and cereals. Thorough chewing not only gives valuable exercise to the teeth, but, by grinding up these foods thoroughly, makes them easier for the stomach to digest; and, by mixing them well with the saliva, enables it to change the starch into sugar. Meats, fish, eggs, cheese, etc., do not need to be mixed with the saliva, nor to be ground so fine for easy digestion in the stomach, and hence do not require such thorough chewing, though it is better to make a rule of chewing all food well. We can exercise our teeth also by eating plenty of foods that require a good deal of chewing, especially the crusts of bread, and vegetables such as corn, celery, lettuce, nuts, parched grains, and popcorn.

It is most important to keep the nasal passages clear and free, and the teeth sound and regular by proper dental attention, so that the jaws will grow properly, and each tooth will strike squarely against its fellow in the opposite jaw, and both jaws fit snugly and closely to each other, making the bite firm and clean, and the grinding close and vigorous. If we are mouth-breathers, our jaws will grow out of shape, so that our teeth are crowded and irregular and do not meet each other properly in chewing. Pressure upon the roots of the teeth, from meeting their fellows of the opposite jaw in firm, vigorous mastication, is one of the most important means of keeping them sound and healthy. Whenever a tooth becomes idle and useless, from failing to meet its fellow tooth in the jaw above or below properly, or from having no fellow tooth to meet, it is very likely to begin to decay.

The next important thing in keeping the teeth healthy is to keep them thoroughly clean. The greatest enemies of our teeth are the acids that form in the scraps of food that are left between them after eating. Meats are not so dangerous in this regard as starches and sugars, because the fluids resulting from their decay are alkaline instead of acid; but it is best to keep the teeth clear of scraps of all kinds. This can best be done by the moderate and gentle use of a quill, or rolled wooden tooth-pick, followed by a thorough brushing after each meal with a rather stiff, firm brush. Then use floss-silk, or linen or rubber threads to "saw" out such pieces as have lodged between the teeth.

This brushing should be given, not merely to the teeth, but to the entire surface of the gums as well; for, as we have seen, it is the gums that make or spoil the health of the teeth, and they, like all other parts of the body, require plenty of exercise and pressure in order to keep them healthy. In the early days of man, when he had no knives and gnawed his meat directly off the bones, and when he cracked nuts and ground all his grain with his teeth, the gums got an abundance of pressure and friction and were kept firm and healthy and red; but now that we take out the bones of the meat and stew or hash it, have all our grain ground, and strip off all the husks of our vegetables and skins of our fruits, though we have made our food much more digestible, we have robbed our gums of a great deal of valuable friction and exercise.

The most practical way to make up for this is by vigorous massage and scrubbing with a tooth-brush for five minutes at least three times a day. It will hurt and even make the gums bleed at first; but you will be surprised how quickly they will get used to it, so that it will become positively enjoyable.

It is good to use some cleansing alkaline powder upon the brush. The old-fashioned precipitated chalk, which makes the bulk of most tooth powders, is very good; but an equally good and much cheaper and simpler one is ordinary baking soda, or saleratus, though this will make the gums smart a little at first. Any powder that contains pumice-stone, cuttle-fish bone, charcoal, or gritty substances of any sort, as many unfortunately do, is injurious, because these scratch the enamel of the teeth and give the acids in the mouth a chink through which they may begin to attack the softer dentine underneath the "glaze" of enamel.

Antiseptic powders and washes, while widely advertised, are not of much practical value, except for temporary use when you have an abscess in your gums, or your teeth are in very bad condition. It is almost impossible to get them strong enough to have any real effect in checking putrefaction of the food or diseases of the gums, without making them too irritating or poisonous. If you keep the gums and teeth well brushed and healthy, you will need no antiseptics.

Not only should the teeth be kept thoroughly clean and sweet for their own sake, but also for the sake of the stomach and the health of the blood and the whole body. The mouth, being continually moist and warm and full of chinks and pockets, furnishes an ideal breeding ground for all kinds of germs; and the average, uncleansed human mouth will be found to contain regularly more than thirty different species of germs, each numbering its millions! Among them may sometimes be found the germs of serious diseases such as pneumonia, diphtheria, and blood-poisoning, just waiting, as it were, their opportunity to attack the body. In fact, a dirty, neglected mouth is one of the commonest causes of disease.

CHAPTER XXVI

INFECTIONS, AND HOW TO AVOID THEM

What Causes Disease. The commonest and most dangerous accident that is likely to happen to you is to catch some disease. Fortunately, however, this is an accident that is as preventable as it is common. Indeed, if everybody would help the Board of Health in its fight against the spread of the common "catchable" diseases, these diseases could soon be wiped out of existence. Every one of them is due to dirt of some sort; and absolute cleanness would do away with them altogether.

Diseases that are "catching," or will spread from one person to another, are called infections; and all of them, as might be supposed from their power of spreading, are due to tiny living particles, called germs--so tiny that they cannot be seen except under a powerful microscope. Nine-tenths of these disease germs are little plants of the same class as the moulds that grow upon cheese or stale bread, and are called bacteria, or bacilli. The different kinds of bacteria, or bacilli, are usually named after the diseases they produce, or else after the scientists who discovered them. For instance, the germ that causes typhoid fever is called the bacillus typhosus; that which causes tuberculosis is called the bacillus tuberculosis; while the germ of diphtheria known as the Klebs-Loeffler bacillus, after the two men who discovered it.

A few kinds of disease germs belong to the animal kingdom, though all germs are so tiny that you would have to have a very powerful microscope to tell the difference between the animal germs and the bacilli, or little plants. Most of these animal germs are called protozoa and cause diseases found in, or near, the tropics, like malaria and the terrible "sleeping sickness" of Africa. Smallpox, yellow fever, and hydrophobia--the disease that results from the bite of a mad dog--are also probably due to animal germs.

So far as prevention is concerned, however, it makes practically little difference whether infectious diseases are due to an animal or a vegetable germ, or to one bacillus or another. They all have two things in common: they can be spread only by the touch of an infected person, and "touch" includes breath,--indeed "by touch" is the meaning of both infectious and contagious; and they can all be prevented by the strictest cleanness, or killed by various poisons known as germicides ("germ-killers"), or disinfectants. Most of these germicides are, unfortunately, poisonous to us as well; for, as you will remember, our bodies are made up of masses of tiny animal cells, not unlike the animal germs. Most of the germicides, therefore, have to be used against germs while they are outside of our bodies.

Scripture says that "a man's foes shall be they of his own household," and this is true of disease germs. They grow and flourish--and, so far as history tells us, the diseases they cause seem to have started--only where people are crowded together in huts or houses, breathing one another's breaths and one another's perspiration, and drinking one another's waste substances in the well water. This fact has, however, its encouraging side; for, since this habit of crowding together, which we call civilization, or "citification," has caused and keeps causing these diseases, it can also cure them and prevent their spread if all the people will fight them in dead earnest. No amount of money, or of time, that a town or a county can spend in stamping out these infectious diseases would be wasted. Indeed, every penny of it would be a good investment; for, taken together, they cause at least half, and probably nearly two-thirds, of all deaths. Not only so, but most of the so-called chronic diseases of the heart, kidneys, lungs, bones, and brain are due to the after-effects of their toxins, or poisons.

How Disease Germs Grow and Spread. But perhaps you will ask, "If these bacteria and protozoa are so tiny that we have to use a microscope, and one of the most powerful made, in order even to see them, how is it that they can overrun our whole body and produce such dangerous fevers and so many deaths?" The answer is simply, "Because there are so many millions of them; and because they breed, or multiply, at such a tremendously rapid rate." When one of these little bacilli breeds, it doesn't take time to form buds and flowers and seeds, like other plants, or even the trouble to lay eggs like an insect or a bird, but simply stretches itself out a little longer, pinches itself in two, and makes of each half a new bacillus.

This is known as fission or "splitting," and is of interest because this is the way in which the little cells that make up our own bodies increase in number; as, for instance, when a muscle is growing and enlarging under exercise, or when more of the white blood cells are needed to fight some disease. Remember that we and the disease germs are both cells; and that, if they are numbered by millions, we are by billions; and that we are made up of far the older and the tougher cells of the two. Except in a few of the most virulent and deadly of fevers, like the famous "Black Death," or bubonic plague, and lock-jaw, or tetanus, ninety-five times out of a hundred when disease germs get into our bodies, it is our bodies that eat up the germs instead of the germs our bodies. Keep away from disease germs all that you reasonably and possibly can; but don't forget that the best protection against infectious diseases, in the long run, is a strong, vigorous, healthy body that can literally "eat them alive."

Grow that kind of body, keep it perfectly clean inside and out, and you have little need to fear fevers, or indeed any other kind of disease; for you will live until you are old enough to die--and then you'll want to, just as you want to go to sleep when you are tired. Remember that this fight against the fevers is a winning fight, this study of disease germs a cheering and encouraging one, because it will end in our conquering them, not merely nine times out of ten, but ninety-nine times out of a hundred.

We are not making this fight just to escape death; what we are fighting for is to live out a full, useful, and happy life. And we already have five chances to one of gaining this, and the chances are improving every year; for science has already raised the average length of life from barely twenty years to over forty. Broadly speaking, if you will keep away from every one whom you know to have an infectious disease; wash your hands always before you eat, or put anything into your mouth; keep your fingers, pencils, pennies, and pins out of your mouth,--where they don't belong; live and play in the open air as much as possible and keep your windows well open day and night, you will avoid nine-tenths of the risks from germs and the dangers that they bring in their wake.

Children's Diseases. We have already studied two of the greatest and most dangerous diseases, and the way to conquer them--tuberculosis, or consumption, in the chapter on the lungs; and typhoid fever, in the chapter on our drink. One of the next most important groups of "catching" diseases--important because, though very mild, they are so exceedingly common,--is that known as the "diseases of childhood," or "diseases of infancy" because they are most likely to occur in childhood. So common are they that you know their names almost as well as you know your own--measles, mumps, whooping cough, scarlet fever, and chicken-pox. Though they are in no way related to one another, so far as we know (indeed, the precise germs that cause two of them--measles and scarlet fever--have not yet positively been determined), yet they can be practically taken together, because they are all spread in much the same way, they all begin with much the same sort of sneezing and inflammation of the nose and throat, they can all be prevented by the same means, and, if properly taken care of, they result in complete recovery ninety-five times out of a hundred.

Statistics for the population of the old City of New York. The chart shows a decrease from 95 out of every 1,000 in 1891-92 to 48 out of every 1,000 in 1909. This is due very largely to the careful methods of prevention enforced by the Board of Health, especially the inspection of milk.]

Any child who has sneezing, running at the nose or eyes, sore throat, or cough, especially with headache or backache, a flushed face and feverishness, ought to be kept at home from school and placed in a well-ventilated, well-lighted room by himself for a day or two, until it can be seen whether he has one of these children's diseases, or only a common cold. If it turns out to be measles, scarlet fever, or whooping cough, he should then be kept entirely away from other children in a separate room, or, where that is impossible, in a special hospital or ward for the purpose; he should be kept in bed and given such remedies as the doctor may advise. Then no one else will catch the disease from him; and within from two to five weeks, he will be well again. The most important thing is not to let him get up and begin to run about, or expose himself, too soon; five times as many deaths are caused by taking cold, or becoming over-tired, or by injudicious eating, during recovery after measles, scarlet fever, and whooping cough, as by the disease itself. This one caution will serve two purposes; for, as a sick child's breath, and the scales from his skin, and what he coughs out from his mouth and nose are full of germs, and will give the disease to other children from two to four weeks after the fever has left him, he ought to be kept by himself--"in quarantine," as we say--for this length of time, which is just about the period needed to protect him from the dangers of relapse or taking cold. Boards of Health fix this period of quarantine by law and put a colored placard on the house to warn others of the danger of infection.

Colds and Sore Throats. A milder and even more common kind of infection is that known as common colds. These, as shown by their name, were once supposed to be due to exposure to cold air, or drafts, or to becoming wet or chilled. But, while a few of them are so caused, at least eight, and probably nine, out of ten are due to germs caught from somebody else. They are never caught in the open air and very seldom in cold, pure fresh air of any sort, but almost always in the hot, foul, stuffy, twice-breathed air of bedrooms, schoolrooms, churches, theatres, halls, sleeping cars, etc. The colds, for instance, that you catch when traveling, are usually due not to drafts or damp sheets, but to the crop of cold germs left behind by the last victim.

You have probably known of colds that have run through a family or a school or a shop. It is well worth trying to keep away from the infection of colds, because not only is their coughing and sore throat and hoarseness and running at the nose very disagreeable and uncomfortable, but they may cause almost as many different kinds of serious troubles in heart, kidneys, and nervous system as any of the other infections. In fact, they probably cause more than any other, because they are at least ten times as common and frequent. For instance, many cases of rheumatism, or rheumatic fever, come after attacks in the nose and throat, which cannot be distinguished from a common cold or ordinary tonsilitis. Indeed, it is more than probable that one of the ten or a dozen different germs that may get into your nose or throat and give you a cold, is the germ that causes rheumatism. At all events, it would be fairly safe to say, "No colds, no rheumatism."

Whenever you have a cold, keep away from everybody that you possibly can and stay at home from school or business for a day or two. You will do no good to yourself or others, working in that condition; and you may infect a dozen others. If you find anyone in your class or room or shop, sneezing or coughing or running at the nose, report him to your teacher or foreman; and if he won't send him home, keep away from him as much as possible.

Diphtheria. Another common and serious disease, until quite recently very fatal, is diphtheria. This is caused by getting into your mouth or nose the germs from another case of the disease. This disease also is most likely to occur in childhood, though it may attack a person of any age, and is always serious. It may be prevented from spreading by keeping children who have it shut up in rooms, or wards, by themselves and keeping all other children away from them, or from their nurses or those who have anything to do with them. Up to about thirty years ago, it was one of the deadliest and most terrible diseases that we had anything to do with. We knew absolutely nothing that would cure it, or even check its course; and nearly half of the children attacked by it died.

About that time, however, two scientists, Klebs and Loeffler, discovered that, by taking some of the membrane, or tough growth that forms in the throat in this disease, and by rubbing it over a plate of gelatin jelly, they could grow on that gelatin a particular kind of germ. This germ, or bacillus, they then put into the throats of guinea pigs, and found that it would give them diphtheria.

This is the way disease germs are discovered, or, as we say, identified; but of course this did not give at once any remedy for the disease. Scientists soon found, however, that, if a very small number of these bacilli were put into a guinea pig's throat, it would have diphtheria, but in a very mild form. If, when it had recovered, it was again infected, it would stand a much larger dose of the bacilli without harm. This made them suspect that some substance had been formed in the guinea-pig's blood that killed the bacillus or worked against its toxin, or poison; and soon, to their delight, they succeeded in finding this substance, which they called antitoxin (meaning "against poison"). Then came the idea that if they could only get enough of this antitoxin, and inject it into the blood of a child who had diphtheria, it might cure the disease. A guinea pig is such a tiny animal that the amount of antitoxin which it could form would be far too small to cure a man, or even a child. So larger animals were taken; and it was finally found that the largest and strongest of our domestic animals, the horse, would, if the diphtheria germs were injected into its blood, make such large amounts of antitoxin that merely by drawing a quart or two of the blood--and closing up the vein again--enough antitoxin could be got to cure fifty or a hundred children of diphtheria. This treatment has not the slightest harmful effect upon the horse. The pain of injecting is only like sticking a pin through the skin, while the pain of bleeding is no greater than cutting your finger. There are now at our great manufacturing laboratories whole stables full of horses, for the production of this wonderful remedy.

Statistics from the City of New York. Antitoxin was used largely from 1893-95, during which time there was a steady decrease (from 60% to 30%) in the death-rate. After the Board of Health took up the matter, furnishing antitoxin without cost, the death-rate continued to decrease to less than 10% of the total number of cases, in 1909.]

With this remedy, our entire feeling toward diphtheria is changed. Instead of dreading it above all things, we know now, from hundreds of thousands of cures, that, if a case is seen on the first day of the disease, and this antitoxin injected with a hypodermic needle, it is almost certain that the patient will recover; not more than two or three cases out of a hundred will fail. If the case is seen and treated on the second day, all but four or five out of a hundred will recover; and if on the third day, all but ten. In fact, the average death rate of diphtheria has been cut down now from forty-five per cent to about six per cent.

We now have antitoxins, or vaccines, for blood-poisoning; for typhoid fever; for one of the forms of rheumatism; for boils; for the terrible cerebro-spinal meningitis, or "spotted fever"; and for tetanus, or lock-jaw. And every year there are one or two other diseases added to the list of those that have been conquered in this way.

None of these vaccines is so powerful, or so certain in its effects, as the diphtheria antitoxin. But they are very helpful already; and some of them, particularly the typhoid vaccine, are of great value in preventing the attack of the disease, as small doses of it given to persons who have been exposed to the infection, or are obliged to drink infected water, as in traveling or in war, very greatly lessen their chances of catching the disease.

Vaccination, the Great Cure for Smallpox. Another valuable means of preventing disease by means of its germs is by putting very small doses of the germs into a patient's body, so that they will give him a very mild attack of the disease, and cause the production in his blood of such large amounts of antitoxin that he will no longer be liable to an attack of the violent, or dangerous, form of the disease. Vaccines, for this purpose, usually consist either of a very small number of the disease germs, or of a group of them, which have been made to grow upon a very poor soil or have been chilled or heated so as to destroy their vitality or kill them outright. When these dead, or half-dead, bacilli are injected into the system, they stir up the body to produce promptly large amounts of its antitoxin. In some cases the reaction is so prompt and so vigorous that the antitoxin is produced almost without any discomfort, or disturbance, and the patient scarcely knows anything about it. In others there will be a slight degree of feverishness, with perhaps a little headache, and a few days, or hours, of discomfort. When this has passed, then the individual is protected against that disease for a period varying from a few months to as long as seven or eight years, or even for life.

The best-known and oldest illustration of the use of these vaccines is that of smallpox. A little more than a hundred years ago, an English country doctor by the name of Jenner discovered that the cows in his district suffered from a disease accompanied by irritation upon their skins and udders, which was known as "cowpox." The dairymaids who milked these cows caught this disease, which was exceedingly mild and was all over within four or five days; but after that the maids would not take smallpox, or, as we say, were immune against it. Smallpox at that time was as common as measles is now. Nearly one-fourth of the whole population of Europe was pock-marked, and over half the inmates in the blind asylums had been made blind by smallpox. So common was it that it was quite customary to take the infectious matter from the pocks upon the skin of a mild case and inoculate children with it, so as to give them the disease in mild form and thus protect them against a severe, or fatal, attack; just as in country districts, a few years ago, some parents would expose their children to measles when it happened to be a mild form, so as to "have it over with."

It occurred to Dr. Jenner that if this inoculation with cowpox would protect these milkmaids, it would be an infinitely safer thing to use to protect children than even the mildest known form of inoculation. So he tried it upon two or three of his child patients, after explaining the situation to their parents, and was perfectly delighted when, a few months afterward, these children happened to be exposed to a severe case of smallpox and entirely escaped catching the disease. This was the beginning of what we now call vaccination.

The germ of cowpox, which is believed to be either the cow or horse variety of human smallpox, is cultivated upon healthy calves. The matter formed upon their skin is collected with the greatest care; and this is rubbed, or scraped, into the arm of the child. It is a perfectly safe and harmless cure; and although it has been done millions of times, never has there been more than one death from it in 10,000 cases. In a little over a hundred years it has reduced smallpox from the commonest and most fatal of all diseases to one of the rarest. But in every country in the world into which vaccination has not been introduced, smallpox rages as commonly and as fatally as ever. For instance, between 1893 and 1898 in Russia, where a large share of the people are unvaccinated, 275,000 deaths occurred from smallpox; in Spain, where the same condition exists, 24,000. In Germany, on the other hand, where vaccination is practically universal, there were in the same period only 287 deaths--1/1000 as many as in Russia; and in England, only a slightly greater number.

Another illustration, which comes closer home, is that of the Philippine Islands. Before they were annexed by the United States, vaccination was rare, and thousands of deaths from smallpox occurred every year. In 1897, after the people had been thoroughly vaccinated, there was not a single death from this cause in the whole of the Islands.

This discovery of Jenner's was most fortunate; for vaccination remains until this day absolutely the only remedy of any value whatever that we possess against smallpox.

Quarantine, inoculation, improvement of living and sanitary conditions, the use of drugs and medicines of all sorts other than vaccination, have no effect whatever upon either the spread or the fatality of the disease. The author, when State Health Officer of Oregon, saw the disease break out in a highly-civilized, well-fed, well-housed community, and kill eleven out of thirty-three people attacked, just as it would have done in the "Dark Ages." Not one of the cases that died had been vaccinated; and, with but one exception (and in this the proof of vaccination was imperfect), every vaccinated case recovered. Vaccination will usually protect for from five to ten years; then it is advisable to be re-vaccinated, and in six to eight years more, another vaccination should be attempted. This third vaccination will usually not "take," for the reason that two successful vaccinations will usually protect for life.

Unexpected as it may seem, vaccination is not only a preventive of smallpox, but a cure for it. The reason being that vaccinia, the disease resulting from successful vaccination, being far milder than smallpox, runs its course more quickly,--taking only two days to develop,--while smallpox requires anywhere from seven to twenty days to develop after the patient has been infected, or exposed. So, if anyone who has been exposed to smallpox is vaccinated any time within a week after exposure, the vaccine will take hold first, and the patient will have either simple vaccinia, with its trifling headache and fever, or else a very mild form of smallpox.

Some persons object to having children deliberately infected with even the mildest sort of disease; but this is infinitely better than to allow, as was the case before vaccination, from one-fourth to one-fifth of them to be killed, twenty-five per cent of them to be pock-marked, and ten per cent of them to be blinded by this terrible disease. So far as any after-effects of vaccination are concerned, careful investigation of hundreds of thousands of cases has clearly shown that it is not so dangerous as a common cold in the head.

Infantile Paralysis. Another disease that has been unpleasantly famous of late is also caused and spread by a germ. This is a form of laming or crippling of certain muscles in childhood known as infantile paralysis. It is not a common disease, though during the last two years there has been an epidemic of it in the United States, especially in New York and Massachusetts. The only things of importance for you to know about it are that it begins, like the other infections, with headache, fever, and usually with "snuffles" or slight sore throat, or an attack of indigestion; and that its germ is probably spread by being sneezed or coughed into the air from the noses and throats of the children who have it, and breathed in by well children. The best known preventive of serious results from this disease is the same as in the rest of infectious diseases, namely, rest in bed, away from all other children, which at the same time stops the spread of it. It furnishes one more reason why all children having the "snuffles" and sore throat with fever and headache should be kept away from school and promptly put to bed and kept there until they are better.

The reason why the disease produces paralysis is that its germs specially attack the spinal cord, so as to destroy the roots of the nerves going to the muscles. Unless the harm done to the spinal cord is very severe, other muscles of the arm or the leg can very often be trained to take the place and to do the work of the paralyzed muscles, so that while the limb will not be so strong as before, it will still be quite useful.

Malaria. Practically the only disease due to animal germs, which is sufficiently common in temperate or even subtropical regions to be of interest to us, is malaria, better known perhaps as ague, or "chills-and-fever." This disease has always been associated with swamps and damp marshy places and the fogs and mists that rise from them; indeed its name, mal-aria, is simply the Italian words for "bad air." It is commonest in country districts as compared with towns, in the South as compared with the North, and on the frontier, and usually almost disappears when all the ponds and swamps in a district are drained and turned into cultivated land or meadows.

About four hundred years ago, the Spanish conquerors of America were fortunate enough to discover that the natives of Peru had a bitter, reddish bark, which, when powdered or made into a strong tea, would cure ague. This, known first as "Peruvian bark," was introduced into Europe by the intelligent and far-sighted Spanish Countess of Chincon; and, as she richly deserved, her name became attached to it--first softened to "cinchona" and later hardened to the now famous "quinine." But for this drug, the settlement of much of America would have been impossible. The climate of the whole of the Mississippi Valley and of the South would have been fatal to white men without its aid.

But although we knew that we could both break up and prevent malaria by doses of quinine large enough to make the head ring, we knew nothing about the cause--save that it was always associated with swamps and marshy places--until about forty years ago a French army surgeon, Laveran, discovered in the red corpuscles of the blood of malaria patients, a little animal germ, which has since borne his name. This, being an animal germ, naturally would not grow or live like a plant-germ and must have been carried into the human body by the bite of some other animal. The only animals that bite us often enough to transmit such a disease are insects of different sorts; and, as biting insects are commonly found flying around swamps, suspicion very quickly settled upon the mosquito.

By a brilliant series of investigations by French, Italian, English, and American scientists, the malaria germ was discovered in the body of the mosquito, and was transmitted by its bite to birds and animals. Then a score or more of eager students and doctors in different parts of the world offered themselves for experiment--allowed themselves to be bitten by infected mosquitoes, and within ten days developed malaria. At first sight, this discovery was not very encouraging; for to exterminate mosquitoes appeared to be as hopeful a task as to sweep back the Atlantic tides with a broom. But luckily it was soon found that the common piping, or singing, mosquito (called from his voice Culex pipiens) could not carry the disease, but only one rather rare kind of mosquito (the Anopheles), which is found only one-fiftieth as commonly as the ordinary mosquito. It was further found that these malaria-bearing mosquitoes could breed only in small puddles, or pools, that were either permanent or present six months out of the year, and that did not communicate with, or drain into, any stream through which fish could enter them. Fish are a deadly enemy of the mosquito and devour him in the stage between the egg and the growth of his wings, when he lives in water as a little whitish worm, such as you may have seen wriggling in a rain-barrel.

It was found that by hunting out a dozen or twenty little pools of this sort in the neighborhood of a town full of malaria, and filling them up, or draining them, or pouring kerosene over the surface of the water, the spread of the malaria in the town could be stopped and wiped out absolutely. This has been accomplished even in such frightfully malarial districts as the Panama Canal Zone, and the west coast of Africa, whose famous "jungle fever" has prevented white men from getting a foothold upon it for fifteen hundred years. Since the young mosquitoes, in the form of wrigglers, or larv? cannot grow except in still water, draining the pools kills them; and, as they must come to the surface of the water to breathe, pouring crude petroleum over the water--the oil floating on the surface and making a film--chokes them.

The common garden mosquito, while not dangerous, is decidedly a nuisance and can be exterminated in the same way--by draining the swamps and pools, or by flooding them with crude petroleum,--or by draining swamps or pools into fresh-water ponds and then putting minnows or other fish into these ponds. There is no reason why any community calling itself civilized should submit to be tormented by mosquitoes if it will spend the few hundred, or the thousand, dollars necessary to wipe them out. It is prophesied that the use of quinine will soon become as rare as it is now common, because malaria will be wiped out by the prevention of the mosquito.

Disinfectants. So far we have been considering how to attack the germs after they have got into our bodies, or to prevent them from spreading from one patient to another; but there is still another way in which they may be attacked, and that is by killing, or poisoning them, outside the body. This process is generally known as disinfection, and is carried out either by baking, boiling, or steaming, or by the use of strongly poisonous fluids or gases, known as disinfectants.

While fortunately none of these disease germs can breed, or reproduce their kind, outside the human body, and while comparatively few of them live very long outside the human body, they may, if mixed with food or caught upon clothing, hangings, walls, or floors, remain in a sort of torpid, but still infectious, condition for weeks or even months. Consequently, it has become the custom to take all the bedding, clothing, carpets, curtains, etc., that have touched a patient suffering from a contagious disease, or have been in the room with him, and also any books that he may have handled, any pens or pencils that he may have used, and either destroy them, or bake, boil, or fumigate them with some strong germicidal, or disinfectant, vapor.

The photograph shows work done in the Panama Canal Zone. The swamp has already been drained by ditches, and the work of destroying the larv?is being completed by the use of oil.]

This is usually done by closing up tightly the sick-room, putting into it all clothing, bedding, pictures, books, hangings, and other articles used during the illness (except wash-goods, which, of course, can be sterilized by thorough boiling; and dishes and table utensils, which also can be scalded and boiled); draping the carpet over chairs so as to expose it on all sides, opening closets and drawers, and then filling the room full of some strong germ-destroying fumes.

One of the best disinfectants, and the one now most commonly used by boards of health for this purpose, is formaldehyde--a pungent, irritating gas, which is an exceedingly powerful germ-destroyer. This, for convenience in handling is usually dissolved, or forced into water, which takes up about half its bulk; and the solution is then known as formalin.

When formalin is poured into an open dish, it rapidly evaporates, or gives up its gas; and, if it be gently heated, this will be thrown off in such quantities as to completely fill the room and penetrate every crevice of it, and every fold of the clothing or hangings. One pound, or pint, of formalin will furnish vapor enough to disinfect a room eight feet square and eight feet high, so the amount for a given room can thus be calculated. The formalin vapor will attack germs much more vigorously and certainly if it be mixed with water vapor, or steam; so it is usually best either to boil a large kettle of water in the room for half an hour or more, so as to fill the air with steam, before putting in the formalin, or to use a combination evaporator with a lamp underneath it, which will give off both formalin and steam. This, if lighted and placed on a dish in the centre of a wash-tub or a large dishpan, with two or three inches of water in the bottom of it, can be put into the room and left burning until it goes out of its own accord.

Another very good method is to take a pan, or basin, with the required amount of formalin (not more than an inch or two inches deep) in the bottom of it, get everything ready with doors and windows fastened tight and strips of paper pasted across the cracks, pour quickly over the formalin some permanganate of potash (about a quarter of a pound to each pound of formalin), and then bolt for the door as quickly as possible to avoid suffocation. The resulting boiling up, or effervescence, will throw off quantities of formaldehyde gas so quickly as to drive it into every cranny and completely through clothing, bedding, etc. The room should be left closed up tightly for from twelve to thirty-six hours, when it can be opened--only be careful how you go into it, first sniffing two or three times to be sure that all the gas has leaked out, or holding your breath till you can get the windows open; and in a few hours the room will be ready for use again.

Another older and much less expensive disinfectant for this purpose is common sulphur. From one to three pounds of this, according to the size of the room, is burned by a specially prepared lamp in a pan placed in the centre of a dishpan of water, and the vapor thus made is a very powerful disinfectant. This, however, is a very poisonous and suffocating gas (as you will remember if you have ever strangled on the fumes of an old-fashioned sulphur match) and, compared with formalin, is nearly five times as poisonous to human beings, or animals, and not half so much so to the germs. Where formalin cannot be secured, sulphur is very effective; but its only merit compared with formalin is that it is cheaper, and more destructive to animal parasites and vermin such as bugs, cockroaches, mice, rats, etc., when these happen to be present. Formalin has the additional advantage of not tarnishing metal surfaces, as sulphur does.

It is a good thing for every household and every schoolroom to have a bottle of formalin on hand, so that you may sniff the vapor of it into your nostrils and throat if you think you have been exposed to a cold, or other infectious disease, or make a solution with which to wash your hands, handkerchiefs, pencils, etc., after touching any dirt likely to contain infection. Half a teaspoonful in a bowl of water is enough for this. A saucerful of it placed in an air-tight box, or cabinet, will make a disinfecting chamber in which pencils, books, etc., can be placed over night; and a teaspoonful of it in a quart of water will make an actively germ-destroying solution, which can be used to soak clothing, clean out bedroom utensils, or pour down sinks, toilets, or drains. It is a good thing also to pour a few teaspoonfuls occasionally on the floor of the closets in which your shoes, trousers, dresses, and other outdoor clothing are kept, as these are quite likely to be contaminated by germs from the dust and dirt of the streets.

Formalin is one of the best and safest general disinfectants to use. Its advantages are, that it is nearly ten times as powerful a germicide as carbolic acid, or even corrosive sublimate, so that it may be used in a solution so weak as to be practically non-poisonous to human beings. It is so violently irritating to lips, tongue, and nostrils as to make it almost impossible for even a child to swallow it, while the amount that would be absorbed if taken into the mouth and spit out again would be practically harmless, so far as danger to life is concerned, though it would blister the lips and tongue.

Bacteria, our Best Friends. While, naturally, the bacteria that do us harm by producing disease are the ones that have attracted our keenest attention and that we talk about most, it must never be forgotten that they form only a very, very small part of the total number of bacteria, or germs. These tiny little germs swarm everywhere; and the mere fact that we find bacteria in any place, or in any substance, is no proof whatever that we are in danger of catching some disease there.

All our farm and garden soil, for instance, is full of bacteria that not only are harmless, but give that soil all its richness, or fertility. If you were to take a shovelful of rich garden earth and bake it in an oven, so as to destroy absolutely all bacteria in it, you would have spoiled it so that seeds would scarcely grow in it, and it would not produce a good crop of anything. These little bacteria, sometimes called the soil-bacteria, or bacteria of decay, swarm in all kinds of dead vegetable and animal matter, such as leaves, roots, fruits, bodies of animals, fishes, and insects, and cause them to decay or break down and melt away. In doing this they produce waste substances, particularly those that contain ammonia, or nitrates, or some other form of nitrogen, which are necessary for the growth of plants or crops.

This is why soil can be made richer by scattering over it and plowing into it manure, waste from slaughter houses, or any other kind of decaying animal or vegetable matter. This is promptly attacked by the bacteria of the soil and turned into these easily soluble plant foods. The roots of the plants grown in the soil could no more take this food directly from dead leaves or manure than you could live on sawdust or cocoanut matting.

So, if it were not for these bacteria, or lower plants, there could be no higher, or green, plants. As animals live either upon these green plants, such as grass and grains, or upon the flesh of other animals that live upon plants, we can see that without the bacteria there would be no animal life, not even man. No bacteria, no higher life. It would be safe to say that, out of every million bacteria in existence, at least 999,999 are not only not harmful but helpful to us.

One large group of bacteria produces the well-known souring of milk; and while this in itself is not especially desirable, yet the milk is still wholesome and practically harmless, and its sourness prevents the growth of a large number of other bacteria whose growth would quickly make it dangerous and poisonous. Many races living in hot countries deliberately sour all the milk directly after milking, by putting sour milk into it, because, when soured, it will keep fairly wholesome for several days, while if not soured it would entirely spoil and become unusable within twenty-four hours.

Another group of bacteria, which float about in the air almost everywhere, are the yeasts, which we harness to our use for the very wholesome and healthful process of bread-making. Millions upon millions of bacteria of different sorts live and grow naturally in our stomachs and intestines; and while they are probably of no special advantage to us, yet at the same time the majority of them are practically, within reasonable limits--not to exceed a few billions or so--harmless.

Insect Pests. One kind of "dirt" that should be avoided with special care is insects of all sorts. No one needs to be told to try to keep a house, or a room, clear of fleas, bed-bugs, or lice; indeed to have these creatures about is considered a mortal disgrace. Not only is their bite very unpleasant, but they may convey a variety of diseases, including plague and blood poisonings of various sorts. But there is another insect pest far commoner and far more dangerous than either fleas or bed-bugs, whose presence we should feel equally ashamed of; and that is the common house fly. This filthy little insect breeds in, and feeds upon, filth, manure, garbage, and dirt of all sorts, and then comes and crawls over our food, falls into our milk, wipes his feet on our sugar and cake, crawls over the baby's face, and makes a general nuisance of himself. Take almost any fly that you can catch, let him crawl over a culture plate of gelatin, put that gelatin away in a warm place, and you will find a perfect flower-garden of germs growing up all over it, following the pattern made by the tracks of his dirty feet. In this garden will be found not "silver bells and cockle shells and pretty maids all in a row," but a choice mixture of typhoid bacilli, pus germs, the germs of putrefaction, tubercle bacilli, and the little seeds which, if planted in our own bodies, would blossom as pneumonia or diphtheria.

The fly is an unmitigated nuisance and should be wiped out. No half-way measures should be considered. Fortunately, this is perfectly possible; for his presence is our own fault and nothing else, as he can lay his eggs and hatch only in piles of dirt and filth found about our own houses, barns, and outbuildings. He is not a wild insect but a domestic one and is practically never found more than a few hundred yards away from some house or barnyard. His favorite place for breeding is in piles of stable manure, especially horse manure; but neglected garbage cans, refuse heaps, piles of dirt and sweepings, decaying matter of all sorts, which are allowed to remain for more than ten days or two weeks at a time, will give him the breeding grounds that he needs.

It takes him about two weeks to hatch and get away from these breeding places; so that if everything of this sort is cleaned up carefully once a week, or if, where manure heaps and garbage dumps have to remain for longer periods, they are sprinkled with arsenic, kerosene, corrosive sublimate, chloride of lime, or carbolic acid, he will perish and disappear as surely as grass will if you wash away the soil in which it grows. The presence of a fly means a dirty house or a dirty yard somewhere, and to discover a fly in your house should be considered a disgrace. Until people are aroused to the need of such cleanliness as will make flies disappear entirely, in most places it will be necessary, as warm weather approaches, to screen all doors and windows, and particularly all boxes, pantries, or refrigerators in which food is kept. If you cannot afford screens, use fly paper. These are all, however, only half-way measures and will give only partial relief. The best prevention of flies is absolute cleanliness. No dirt, no flies.

Dust, a Source of Danger. Dust is an easily recognized form of dirt. It is dangerous in itself and nearly always contains germs of one sort or another mixed in with it. Shops and factories whose processes make much dust are usually very unhealthy for the workers, who are likely to show a high death-rate from consumption.

Dust should be fought and avoided in every possible way. City streets should have good modern pavements,--preferably asphalt or some crude petroleum, or sawmill-waste, "crust," or coating,--which will not make any dust, and which can be washed down every night with a hose. In smaller towns where there is no pavement, dust may be prevented by regular sprinklings during the summer, preferably with some form of crude oil. Two or three full sprinklings of this will keep down the dust for the greater part of the summer.

If these measures are properly carried out, they will prevent most of the dust that accumulates in houses, as nearly all of this blows in through the windows or is carried in on shoes or skirts. When this has once floated in and settled down upon the walls, furniture, or carpets, be very careful how you disturb it; for, as long as it lies there, it will do you no harm, however untidy it may look. The broom and the feather duster and the dry cloth do almost as much harm as they do good; for while they may remove two-thirds of the dust from a room, they drive the other third right into your nose and throat, where the germs it contains can do the most possible harm. Dusting should always be done with a damp cloth; sweeping, with a damp cloth tied over a broom; and, wherever possible, a carpet sweeper, or, better still, a vacuum cleaner, should be used instead of a broom.

Carpets, window curtains, and any hangings that catch dust should be abolished--rugs that can be rolled up and taken out of doors to be shaken and beaten should be used instead; and too many pieces of bric-?brac and ornaments should be avoided. All surfaces of walls, ceilings, and floors should be made as smooth and hard and free from angles, ledges, and projecting lines as possible. The colds usually caught by members of the family during "spring cleaning" are usually due to the swarms of germs stirred up from their peaceful resting places. Let those sleeping germs lie, until you can devise some means of removing them without brushing, or whisking, them straight into your nostrils.

CHAPTER XXVII

ACCIDENTS AND EMERGENCIES

Ordinarily, Accidents are not Serious. Accidents will happen--even in the best regulated families! While taking all reasonable care to avoid them, it is not best to worry too anxiously about the possibility of accidents; for a nervous, fearful state of mind is almost as likely to give rise to them as is a reckless and indifferent one. Fortunately, most accidents, especially with growing boys and girls, are comparatively trifling in their results, and to a considerable extent must simply be reckoned as part of the price that has to be paid for experience, self-control, and skill. To have keen senses, vigorous and elastic muscles, and a clear head, is better protection against accidents than too much caution; it is also the best kind of insurance that can be taken out against their proving serious. The real problem is not so much to avoid accidents as to be ready to meet them promptly, skillfully, and with good judgment when they occur, as they inevitably will. As the old masters of swordsmanship used to teach, "Attack is the best defense."

Luckily, healthy children are as quick as a cat and as tough as sole-leather--if they weren't, the race would have been wiped out centuries ago. Children in their play, on errands, going to and from school, and in excursions through the woods and the fields, run, of course, a great many risks. But in spite of all these dangers, the number of children killed, or even seriously injured, in these "natural" accidents, is not half of one per cent of those who die from disease or bad air or poor food or overwork.

Another cheering thing about accidents is that ninety-nine out of every hundred of them are not serious; and if you are only wise enough to know what to do--and still more what not to do--in taking care of them, you can recover from them safely and quickly. The bodies of healthy children have an astonishing power of repairing themselves. Their bones are not so brittle as those of "grown-ups"; and even when one of them is broken, if properly splinted and dressed, it will heal up in a little more than half the time required by the adult. And wounds and scratches and bruises, if kept perfectly clean, will heal very rapidly.

Probably the commonest of all accidents are cuts and scratches. So common is it for us to "bark" our knuckles, or our shins, or scratch ourselves on nails and splinters and drive pins into ourselves, or let our pocket knives slip and cut our fingers, that, if the human skin had not the most wonderful power of repairing itself,--not merely closing up the cut or the scratch, but making the place "as good as new,"--we should be seamed and lined all over our hands, arms, faces, and limbs like a city map, or scarred and pitted like a tattooed man, before we were fifteen years old. But of course, as you know, the vast majority of cuts and scratches and tears heal perfectly. They hurt when they happen; and they burn, or smart, for a few hours, or hurt, if bumped, for a few days afterward; but they heal soon and are forgotten.

On the other hand, some cuts and scratches will fester and throb and turn to "matter" (pus) and even give you fever and headache and blood poisoning. What makes the difference? It is never the size, or depth, of the scratch or cut itself, but simply the dirt that gets into it afterward. If a cut, or scratch, no matter how deep or ragged, be made with a clean knife-blade or sliver and kept clean afterward, it will never "matter" (suppurate) or cause blood poisoning. So if you know how to keep dirt out of cuts and scratches, you know how to prevent ninety-nine per cent of all the dangers and damage that may come from this sort of accident.

Not more than one cut or scratch in a thousand is deep enough to go down to an artery, so as to cause dangerous bleeding, or to injure an important nerve trunk. So, though no one would by any means advise you to be reckless about getting cut and scratched, yet it is better and safer to run some risk of cuts and scratches in healthy play when young, and learn how to keep them clean, than to grow up pale and flabby-muscled and cowardly.

How to Prevent Infection in Wounds. It is not just dirt that is dangerous,-- although dirt of any sort is a bad thing to get into wounds and should be kept out in every possible way,--but dirt that contains those little vegetable bacteria that we call germs. The dirt most likely to contain these germs--

called pus germs, because they cause pus, or "matter" in a wound--is dirt containing decaying animal or vegetable substances (particularly horse manure, which may contain the tetanus, or lock-jaw germ) and the discharges from wounds, or anything that has come near decayed meat or unhealthy gums or noses or teeth. This is why a cut or scratch made by a knife that has been used for cutting meat, or by a dirty finger-nail, or by the claw of a cat, or by the tooth of a rat, is often likely to fester and "run." Animals like rats and dogs and cats often feed upon badly decayed meat; and hence their teeth, or claws, are quite likely to be smeared with the germs that cause decay, and these will make trouble if they get into a wound.

Fortunately, the care of a cut or scratch is very simple and practically the same in all cases. Just make the wound thoroughly clean and keep it so until it is healed. For a slight clean cut or scratch, a good cleanser is pure water. Hold the hand or foot under the faucet or pump, and let the cool water wash it out thoroughly. If you are sure that the thing you cut it with was clean, let the blood dry on the cut and form a scab over it. If the wound is large, or there is any danger of the water of the well, or tap, having sewage in it (see chapter IX), it is better to boil the water before using it. Unless the blood is spurting in jerks from a cut artery, or bleeding very freely indeed, it is better to let the wound bleed, as this helps to wash out any dirt or germs that have got into it. When the bleeding has stopped, do not put on sticking plaster, because this keeps out the air and keeps in the sweat of the skin surrounding the wound, which is not healthful for the wound, and may also contain some weak pus germs.

If the wound is small, the old-fashioned clean white rag that has been boiled and washed is as good as anything that can be used for a dressing. Tear off a narrow strip from one to two inches wide and as many feet long, according to the position of the wound, roll it round the finger or limb three or four times, and then take a turn round the wrist or nearest joint, to keep the bandage from slipping off. If the wound be likely to keep on oozing blood, put on first a thickness of surgeon's cotton, or prepared cotton-batting, an ounce of which can be purchased for ten cents at any drugstore. This is an excellent dressing, because it not only sucks up, or absorbs any oozing from the wound, but is a perfect filter-protection against germs of all sorts from the outside. Ninety-nine simple wounds out of a hundred dressed in this way will heal promptly and safely without danger of pus, or "matter."

If the wound happens to have been made with a knife or tool that you are not absolutely sure was perfectly clean, or if the wound gets manure or road-dirt or other filth rubbed into it, then it is best to go at once to a doctor and let him give it a thorough antiseptic dressing, which consists of cleaning it out thoroughly with strong remedies, called antiseptics,--which kill the germs, but do not injure living tissues,--and then putting on a germ-proof dressing as before. This is one of the "stitches in time" which will save not only nine, but ninety-nine.

If you have a wound with dirt in it, and cannot reach a doctor, one of the best and safest antiseptics to use is peroxide of hydrogen. This is non-poisonous, and can be poured right into the wound. It will smart and foam, but will clean out and kill most of the germs that are there. Another safe antiseptic is pure alcohol. It is a good thing to have a bottle of one of these in the medicine-closet, or in your "war-bag" when camping out. A package of surgeon's cotton and two or three rolled bandages of old cotton, linen, or gauze also should be on hand.

Dog-bites, rat-bites, or cat-bites should always be dressed by a doctor, or made thoroughly antiseptic, mainly on account of the germs that swarm round the roots of the teeth of these animals, and also because treatment of this sort will prevent hydrophobia--although this danger is a rare and remote one, not more than a few score of deaths from mad-dog bites occurring in the whole United States in a year.

The wonderful progress made by surgery within the last twenty or thirty years has been almost entirely due to two things: first, the discovery of chloroform and ether, which will put patients to sleep, so that they do not feel the pain of even the severest and longest operation; and, second, but even more important, keeping germs of all kinds out of the wound before, during, and after the operation. That sounds simple, but it really takes an immense amount of trouble and pains in the way of baking the dressings; boiling the instruments, and scrubbing with soap, alcohol, hot water, and two or three kinds of antiseptics, or germ-killers, the hands of the surgeon and of the nurse and the body of the patient. How enormous a difference this keeping of the germs out of the wound has made may be gathered from the fact that, while in earlier days, before Lister showed us how to avoid this danger, surgeons used to lose seventy-five per cent of their amputations of the thigh, from pus infection, or blood poisoning, now they can perform a hundred operations of this sort and not lose a single case. We can open into the skull and remove tumors from the brain; open into the chest and remove bullets from the lungs, and even from the heart itself; operate in fact upon any part, or any organ, of the body with almost perfect safety and wonderful success. Whereas, before, two-thirds of the patients so operated upon would die, probably of blood poisoning.

How to Treat Bruises. Bruises are best treated either by holding the injured part under the faucet, or pump, if convenient, or by plunging it into very hot water and holding it there for ten or twelve minutes. Then if the bruise still continues to throb or ache, wrap it up lightly with a bandage of soft, loose cotton or linen cloth, and pour over it a lotion of water containing about one-fourth alcohol until the bandage is soaked, moistening it again as fast as it dries. This is also a useful treatment for wounds that have been made by a fall, or by something blunt and heavy, so that there is bruising as well as cutting. Most of the household applications for wounds or bruises, such as arnica, camphor, witch-hazel, etc., owe their virtues to the five or ten per cent of alcohol they contain, which, by evaporating, cools the wound and relieves inflammation, kills germs and so acts as an antiseptic, and cleans the wound and the skin around it very thoroughly and effectively.

Bruises of all sorts, however, unless very severe, are much safer than cuts or scratches, because they do not break the skin, and consequently no germs can get into the tissues of the blood. Our skin, as you remember, is one of the most wonderful water-proof, germ-proof, hot-and-cold-proof coatings in the world; and as long as it remains unbroken, none but a few of the most virulent disease-germs can get through it into the body.

Boils and Carbuncles, their Cause and their Cure. Boils and carbuncles are almost the only instances in which pus germs can get into the body without some actual cut, tear, or breaking of the skin. They come always from other boils or ulcers or discharging wounds and are caused by the pus germs in these either being rubbed into the skin until it is almost chafed through, or else being driven down into the mouth of one of the hair follicles, or "pores." Here they proceed to grow and form a little gathering, which soon turns to pus; and this stretches the skin and presses upon the sensitive nerves in it so as to cause much pain. The best way to treat them in the beginning is to give a thorough scrubbing with hot water and soap, and then to drop right over the point, or "head," of the gathering two or three drops of a strong antiseptic, like formalin or peroxide or carbolic acid. If this does not check them, then they had better be opened up freely with a sharp knife that has been held in boiling water, or a needle that has been held in a flame until it is red hot and allowed to cool. Then pour peroxide into the opening, put on a light dressing, and keep soaked with alcohol and water, as for a bruise. This evaporating dressing is far superior to the dirty, sticky, germ-breeding poultice. If this does not clear it up within twenty-four hours, go to a doctor and have him treat it antiseptically.

How to Stop Bleeding. If a cut should go deep enough to reach an artery the size of a knitting needle, or larger, then the blood will spurt out in jets. There is then some danger of so much blood being lost as to weaken one. Our blood, however, has a wonderful power of clotting, or clogging, round the mouth of the cut artery, so that the risk of bleeding to death, except from quite a large artery, like that of the thigh, or the armpit, is not very great.

For a wound in the hand or foot, that spurts in this way, it will usually be sufficient to grasp the arm firmly above the wrist or the elbow, or the ankle, as the case may be, with the thumb over the artery, or even to press directly over the wound, until the bleeding stops and the blood is thus given a chance to clot. If the wound is small and deep, like that made by the stab of a knife, or the slip of a chisel, then firm pressure directly over the wound itself with a thumb, or both thumbs, will usually be sufficient to stop the bleeding.

[Illustration: A TOURNIQUET

A stone laid above the cut under the bandage will help to increase the pressure at this point.]

Should, however, the spurting be from an artery like that of the pulse, or from that at the bend of the elbow or the knee, then the best thing to do is to tie quickly a handkerchief or strip of tough cloth loosely around the limb above the wound and, slipping a short stick or bar into the loop, twist upon it, as shown in the picture, until the blood ceases to flow from the wound. It is much better to use a handkerchief or piece of cloth than a cord, because the latter may cut into and damage the tissues, when drawn as tight as is needed to stop the circulation. It is not best to allow a bandage twisted tight enough to stop the circulation--called a tourniquet--to remain tight for more than half an hour at a time, as this may give rise to very dangerous congestion, or serious "blood starvation" of the tissues below it. It should be gently untwisted every half hour until the arm, or limb, below it reddens up again, and then, if the spurting begins, should be tightened as before. There is, however, a good chance that if the cut artery is not too large, the blood will have clotted firmly enough in this time to stop the bleeding; though the tourniquet had better be left on the arm, ready to be tightened at a moment's notice, until the doctor comes.

The Treatment of Burns. Burns require more careful treatment on account of the wide surface of the skin usually destroyed. The layer of the skin that is most alive and most active in the process of repair is the outer layer (the epithelial, or epidermis). A burn, or scald, if at all severe, is likely to destroy almost the entire thickness of this, over its whole extent. This gives both a wide surface for the absorption of pus germs and a long delay in "skinning over," or healing. As the same heat that made the burn has usually destroyed any germs that may be present, it is not necessary to wash or clean a burn, like a wound, unless dirt has been rubbed or sprinkled into it after it has been made. The first thing to be done is to coat it over so as to shut out the air; and this, for a slight burn, can be very well done by dusting it over with baking soda or clean flour or with one of the many dusting, or talc, powders on the market, containing boracic acid, or by laying over the burn a clean cloth soaked in perfectly clean olive oil or vaseline. If the oil or vaseline is not perfectly clean, put it on the top of a stove and heat it thoroughly before using. Dress with soft, clean cotton rag or lint as before, keeping wet with the alcohol lotion (one part of alcohol to eight of water) if there be much pain, or throbbing.

If the burn is deep or the pain at all severe, it is best to call in a doctor, as bad burns are not only agonizingly painful, but also very dangerous on account of the wide, raw surface that they leave open to entrance of pus germs for days and even weeks. Until a doctor can be secured, coat it over with some non-irritating powder or oil, as for lighter burns, or hold it in warm water to exclude the air. Do not try to clean a burn. You only increase the pain of it and probably add to the risk of infection.

If your clothing ever catches fire, wrap yourself up at once in a blanket or rug to smother the flame. Remember that running will supply more air to the flame and cause it to do more damage. If you have nothing at hand in which to wrap yourself, lie down on the floor, or ground, and roll over and over until you have smothered the flame.

What should be Done in the Case of Broken Bones, or Fractures. Broken bones, or fractures, as they are called, are more serious, but fortunately not very common. They should, of course, always be treated by a doctor, to prevent shortening of the limb, or to prevent the bones from growing together at an angle, or in a bad position, so as to interfere with the use of it. Where a doctor cannot readily be had, or the patient has to be taken to him,--as, for instance, where the accident occurs out in the woods,--take two light pieces of board, or two bundles of straight twigs, or two pieces of heavy paper folded fifteen or twenty times--two folded newspapers, for instance--and, wrapping them in cloth or paper, place one on each side of the broken limb, at the same time gently pulling it straight. Then take strips of cloth, or bandage, and bind these splints gently, but firmly and snugly, the length of the limb, so that it cannot be bent in such a way as to make the ends of the bone grate against each other. The patient can then be lifted, or carried, with comparative comfort. Most fractures, or broken bones, in children or young boys or girls, heal very rapidly; and if the limb be properly straightened and splinted by competent hands, it will be practically as good and as strong as before the accident.

Sprains. Sprains are twists or wrenches, of a joint, not severe enough to "put it out," or dislocate it, or to break a bone. A mild sprain is a very trifling affair, but a severe one is exceedingly painful and very slow in healing. The best home treatment for sprains is to hold the injured joint under a stream of cold water for ten or fifteen minutes and then to bandage it firmly and thoroughly, but gently, with a long "figure-of-eight" bandage, wound many times, and to keep this moist with an alcohol lotion. Then keep the limb at rest. If the cold water does not relieve the pain, plunge the joint into water as hot as you can comfortably bear it and keep it there for ten or fifteen minutes, adding fresh hot water to keep up the temperature; then bandage as before.

If the pain should not go down under either of these treatments within six or eight, certainly within ten or twelve, hours, it is far wisest to call a doctor, because severe sprains very often mean the tearing of some important tendon or ligament, and the partial fracture of one of the bones of the joint. Unless these conditions are promptly corrected, you may be laid up for weeks, and even months, and left with a permanently damaged--that is, stiffened--joint. You will often hear it said that a sprain is harder to heal than a fracture; but that kind of sprain usually includes a fracture of some small portion of a bone, which has escaped notice and proper treatment. If the sprain is mild, so that it does not pain you when at rest, then the bandage should be removed every day, and the joint gently rubbed and massaged, and the bandage replaced again. Should there be any one in reach who understands massage, a thorough massaging right after the accident is quite helpful; but no amateur had better attempt it, as unskilled rubbing and stretching are likely to do more harm than good.

What to Do in Case of Poisoning. Poisoning is, fortunately, a rare accident; and the best thing to be done first is practically the same, no matter what poison--whether arsenic, corrosive sublimate, or carbolic acid--has been swallowed. This is to dilute the poison by filling the stomach with warm water and then to bring about vomiting as quickly as possible. This can usually be done by adding a tablespoonful of mustard to each glass of warm water drunk. If this cannot be had, or does not act within a few minutes, then thrusting the finger as far down the throat as it will go, and moving it about so as to tickle the throat, will usually start gagging; or a long feather may be dipped in oil and used in the same way. It is also a good thing to add milk or white of egg or soap to the water, or to mix a little oil or plaster scraped off the wall with it, as these tend to combine with the poison and prevent its being absorbed. If the poison happens to be an acid, like vitriol, then add a tablespoonful or more of baking soda to the hot water; if an alkali, like lye or ammonia, give half a glass of weak vinegar. The main thing, however, is to set up vomiting as quickly as possible.

Another rather frequent and most disagreeable accident, which may happen to you when out in the woods, is poisoning by poison ivy. This is due to the leaves or twigs of a plant, which many of you probably know by sight, touching your hands or face. If you do not happen to know what poison ivy looks like, you had better get some one who knows to point out the shrub to you the next time you go into the woods, and then you should try to keep as far away from it as possible. It is sometimes called poison oak, but both these names are incorrect, as the shrub is really a kind of sumac. It takes its different names because it has the curious habit of either climbing like a vine, when it is called "ivy," or growing erect like a bush, or shrub, when it is called "oak."

All sorts of absurd stories are told about the leaves of the shrub being so poisonous that it is not safe to go within ten feet of it, when the dew is on it, or to walk past it when the wind is blowing from it toward you. But these are pretty nearly pure superstitions, because it has been found that the substance in the leaves or bark of the shrub which poisons the skin is an oil, which is non-volatile, that is to say, will not give off any vapors to the air and, of course, cannot be dissolved in dew or other watery moisture. You must actually touch the leaves in order to be poisoned; but, unfortunately, this is only too easy to do without knowing it when you are scrambling through the woods or hunting for flowers or picking berries.

The remedy for poison ivy is a very simple one, and within the reach of anybody, and is as effective as it is simple. This is a thorough scrubbing of the part poisoned, just as soon as it begins to itch, with a nail-brush and soap and hot water. This makes the skin glow for a little while, but it washes out all the burning and irritating oil and, if used promptly, will usually stop the trouble then and there. It is a good idea if you know that you have touched poison ivy, or even if you have been scrambling about actively in woods or patches of brush where you know that the ivy is common, to give your hands a good washing and scrubbing with sand or mud, if there is no soap at hand, in the first stream or pool that you come to. This will usually wash off the oil before it has had time to get through the natural protective coating of the skin.

Snake-bite is one of the rarest of all accidents and not one-fiftieth as dangerous as usually believed. Not more than one person in twenty bitten by a large rattlesnake will die, and only about two in a hundred bitten by small rattlers or by copperheads. The average poisonous snake of North America cannot kill anything larger than a rabbit, and any medium-sized dog can kill a rattlesnake with perfect safety. Our horror-stricken dread of snakes is chiefly superstition. Of those who die after being bitten by North American snakes, at least half die of acute alcoholic poisoning from the whiskey poured down their throats in pints; and another fourth, from gangrene due to too tight bandaging of the limb to prevent the poison from getting into the circulation, or from pus infections of the wound from cutting it with a dirty knife. Alcohol is as great a delusion and fraud in snake-bite as in everything else; instead of being an antidote, it increases the poisoning by its depressing effect on the heart. If you should be bitten, throw a bandage round the limb, above the bite, and tighten as for a cut artery. Then make with a clean knife two free cuts, about half or three-quarters of an inch deep, through the puncture, one lengthwise and the other crosswise of the limb, and let it bleed freely. Then throw one or, if there be room, two or three other bandages round the limb, three or four inches apart, and tighten gently so as to close the surface veins by the pressure, without shutting off the flow in the arteries. After thirty or forty minutes loosen the first bandage to the same tightness and leave it so unless the heart weakens or faintness is felt, in which case tighten again. If this be done, there isn't one chance in a hundred of any serious result.

How to Avoid Drowning. In case of falling into the water, the chief thing to do is to try to keep calm and to keep your hands below your chin. If you do this and keep paddling, you will swim naturally, just as a puppy or a kitten would, even if you have never learned to swim. It is, however, pretty hard to remember this when you go splash! into the water. Everyone should learn to swim before he is twelve years old; and then in at least nine times out of ten, he will be safe if he fall overboard. Remember that, if you keep your mouth shut and your hands going below your chin, you can keep floating after a fashion, for some time; and in that time the chances are that help will reach you. If you can reach a log or apiece of board or the side of a boat, just cling quietly to that with one hand, and keep paddling with the other. Even if you can get hold of only quite a small limb or pole or piece of a box, by holding one hand on that and paddling with the other and kicking your feet, you will be able to keep floating a long time unless the water be ice cold. If you can manage to keep both your feet splashing on top of the water and both hands going, you can swim several hundred yards.

[Illustration: Pressing out the air in the lungs.

Allowing the lungs to fill themselves.

THE NEW METHOD OF ARTIFICIAL BREATHING

Devised by a celebrated physiologist, Professor Schaefer of Edinburgh, and now being adopted by life-saving stations and crews everywhere.]

You may sometime be called upon to save another person from drowning. In such a case, as in every emergency, a cool head is the chief thing. Make up your mind just what you are going to do before you do anything,--then do it quickly! If no one is near enough to hear your shouts for help, and no boat is at hand, if possible throw, or push, to the one in the water a plank or board or something that will float, and he will instinctively grasp it. If you are thrown into the water with a person that can't swim, grasp his collar or hair, and hold him at arm's length, to prevent his dragging you under, until help arrives, or until you can tow him to safety.

Boys and girls, after they have learned to swim, may well practice rescuing each other, so as to be prepared for such accidents.

Artificial Breathing. The best way to revive a person who has been under water and is apparently drowned, is to turn him right over upon his chest on the ground, or other level surface, turning the face to one side so that the nose and mouth will be clear of the ground. Then, kneeling astride of the legs, as shown in the picture, place both hands on the small of the back and throw your weight forward, so as to press out the air in the lungs. Count three, then swing backward, lifting the hands, and allow the lungs to fill themselves with air for three seconds, then again plunge forward and force the air out of the lungs and again lift your weight and allow the air to flow in for three seconds. Keep up this swinging backward and forward about ten or twelve times a minute. This is the newest and by far the most effective way--in fact the only real way--of keeping up artificial breathing. It is very, very seldom that any one can be revived after he has been under water for more than five minutes,--indeed, after three minutes,--but this method will save all who can possibly be saved.

So perfect a substitute for breathing is it that if any one of you will lie down in this position upon his face, and allow some one else to press up and down on the small of his back after this fashion, ten or twelve times a minute, he will find that, without making any effort of his own to breathe, this pumping will draw enough air into his lungs to keep him quite comfortable for half an hour.

Don't waste any time trying to pour the water out of the lungs. As a matter of fact there is very little there, in drowned people. Don't waste any time in undressing, or warming or rubbing the hands or feet to start the circulation. Get this pendulum pump going and the air blowing in and out of the lungs, and if there is any chance of saving life this will do it; then you can warm and dry and rub the patient at your leisure after he has begun to breathe.

QUESTIONS AND EXERCISES

CHAPTERS

I AND II

1. Look up in a dictionary the words physiology and hygiene. What does each mean? If you can, find the derivation of each. 2. Why should everyone learn about the human body? 3. How is the "man-motor" like an "auto"? Compare the fuel of each. 4. From what source do all the fuels get their force or energy? 5. How do plants get their fuel, or food? 6. What is meant in saying that man takes his food at second, or third, hand? 7. Why do we need a mouth? 8. Does a plant have a mouth? Where? 9. Draw a diagram showing how the food is carried into and throughout the body. 10. Describe the parts of the food tube through which it goes. 11. Tell how the body-motor uses bread as a fuel. How is its form changed before it can be used? 12. What are the salivary glands for? What work is done by their juice? 13. What other juices help to melt the bread? 14. Which foods need the most chewing? 15. How is the food carried down the food tube? 16. What is the appendix? Explain how it sometimes causes trouble. 17. How can you tell the difference between colic and appendicitis? 18. On which side is the appendix located? 19. In what parts of the food tube are (a) starch, (b) meats, (c) fat digested? 20. What causes constipation? How may it be avoided? 21. Is drinking water at meals hurtful? If so, how?

CHAPTER III

1. If we call the body an engine, what is the fuel? what is the smoke? what

are the ashes? 2. Why and how far can we rely upon our natural desires and appetites for food? 3. How should we choose our foods? 4. Name two serious faults that foods may have. 5. Why do we need a variety of foods? 6. What is meant by the term "fuel value of food"? 7. How can we roughly tell to which class a food belongs or what its fuel value is? 8. Why should animal and vegetable foods be used together?

CHAPTER IV

1. Name and describe our most common meats. 2. When is pork a valuable food? 3. Why do we digest it slowly? 4. Why should we eat fish only once or twice a week? 5. What food-stuffs are found in milk? 6. Name some vegetables which contain protein food. 7. In planning a week's diet, how often would you use these vegetables, and why? 8. What is our greatest danger in eating meat? 9. Why is it dangerous to eat highly seasoned stews or hashes? 10. Should cheese be eaten in large amounts at a time? Why? 11. Describe the care taken at a good dairy. 12. Why is this necessary? 13. Why is dirty milk less nourishing than clean milk?

CHAPTER V

1. Explain the name "starch-sugars." To which class of fuel-food might we say that they belong? 2. Why are they cheaper than meat? 3. Why must these foods be ground and cooked? 4. Which is the better food, white or brown bread? Why? 5. Could we live on starch-foods alone? What is the reason of this? 6. In what foods do we find nitrogen? In what, carbon? 7. What is a "complete food"? Name some. 8. Why must the starchy foods be changed in the body into sugar, or glucose? 9. Name three ways by which bread is made "light." 10. What is yeast? 11. How is bread made? 12. Why should it be thoroughly baked? 13. What causes bread to become sour? 14. Name other important starchy foods. 15. Is sugar a valuable food? Why? 16. In what plants do we find it?

CHAPTER VI

1. Why are fats slow of digestion? 2. If they are so valuable as "coal foods," why do we not eat more of them at a meal? 3. Give some reasons for carrying fats as food supply on long voyages and expeditions. 4. In what forms are

they best carried? 5. What makes up the emergency field-ration of the German army, and why? 6. What is the most valuable single fat, and why? 7. Name other fats in common use and describe their effects on digestion. 8. State the food values of bacon. 9. Why should nuts be eaten in moderate quantity only? 10. How do nuts compare in cost (a) with other proteins? (b) with other fats? 11. What is the peanut? 12. Why is it hard to digest? 13. What digestive juices "melt" fats? 14. What is oleomargarine and how does it compare with butter?

CHAPTER VII

1. What is the necessity of fruits and vegetables in our dietary? Why especially in summer? 2. Give some idea of the food value of fruits as compared with bread and meat. 3. Name the most wholesome and useful fruits. 4. What is the food value of bananas? Why is it very important that they be eaten in moderation only? 5. What does (a) boiling and (b) drying do to fruits? 6. Why seal the jars of preserved fruits? 7. Why can you not eat as much jam, at one time, as raw fruit? 8. What disease is caused by scarcity of fresh vegetables or fruits? 9. Name some of the common vegetables and give their fuel values. 10. Why do we need with our meals the lighter green vegetables, although they have little nutritive value? 11. What vegetables contain starch, what sugar, and what digestible protein? 12. In what form is most of the nitrogen of vegetables?

CHAPTER VIII

1. What changes occur in food when it is cooked? Describe some of the changes. 2. What are the advantages of cooking meats and vegetables? 3. Why is it necessary that food should taste good? 4. What has cooking to do with the cost of food? 5. Why is time well spent in cooking food? 6. Describe the different methods of cooking food and tell advantages of each. 7. In what ways can you help make the table attractive and preserve health? 8. In what ways may food be made less digestible and wholesome by cooking? 9. In what way can fried food be made digestible? 10. What is the supposed economy of boiling? 11. Write out a good menu for each meal of the day.

CHAPTER IX

1. Why is water necessary in the body? 2. How does the body take in water other than by drinking it? 3. Why is this water sure to be pure? 4. Why is drinking water likely to be impure? 5. Where and when is water perfectly pure? 6. What are our chief sources of water-supply? 7. What is a well? a spring? a reservoir? 8. Which source of water-supply is safest? 9. What are the dangers of well water? 10. How can they be avoided? 11. What are the dangers of river water? 12. What is a filter and how does it work? 13. What makes water rise in a spring or an artesian well? 14. How may water suspected of being unhealthful be made safe to drink? 15. How is sewage disposed of? 16. How can it be kept out of the drinking water? 17. Why does it pay cities to spend large sums to secure pure water? 18. How can a reservoir be protected? 19. What are the risks of house filters? 20. How do bacteria help us in keeping our water-supply pure? 21. Does your city or town have a central source of water-supply? Where is it? 22. Visit the waterworks of your city or town and describe to the class how the water is obtained, how prepared for use, and how distributed to buildings.

CHAPTER X

1. How can you prove that beverages are not real foods? 2. What is tea? What is coffee? What are chocolate and cocoa? 3. Why are tea and coffee, if stewed, bad for the digestion? 4. Why is it better for you to let these drinks alone? 5. How is alcohol made? 6. How is wine made? beer? cider? whiskey? 7. When does fermentation stop, and for what reason? 8. What is the difference between whiskey and brandy? Why are these the most harmful of these drinks? 9. Explain the effect of alcohol on the digestion. 10. Does it increase the warmth of the body? 11. Does it increase our working power? 12. How is it that at first people thought that alcohol was helpful, when really it was not? 13. What is the effect of alcohol on the nervous system? 14. Can the man who drinks alcohol tell how, or to what extent, it is injuring him? 15. Is alcohol a food or a medicine? 16. How does alcohol usually affect the mind and character? 17. Why is smoking a foolish habit? 18. Why is it harmful for boys? 19. What is nicotine? 20. What proof have we that smoking stunts growth? 21. How is it likely to hinder a boy's career?

CHAPTER XI

1. Where does the real "eating" take place in the body? 2. How is the food

carried to these parts? 3. What does the name "artery" mean? 4. What are veins? 5. If you examine blood under a microscope, what will you find in it? 6. What are the uses of these two kinds of little bodies (corpuscles)? 7. Explain the process of inflammation. 8. Draw a diagram or rough picture showing the route of the blood through the heart and body. Mark the vena cava and the portal vein. 9. What are the capillaries, and what does the name mean? 10. Why do the veins have valves? 11. Explain how the different parts of the heart act, while they are pumping and receiving the blood. 12. How many strokes of the heart-pump are there per minute in a man? a woman? a child? 13. Which part of the heart has the thickest muscle and why? 14. Where are the strongest valves? 15. What blood vessels carry the blood to and from the lungs? 16. What blood vessel carries the blood from the heart over the body? 17. When you press your hand to the left side of your chest, what movement do you feel? 18. Where is the best place to feel the pulse? Why? 19. Which are generally nearer the surface, arteries or veins? Are they near each other? 20. Why does the heart beat faster when you run?

CHAPTER XII

1. Why is it bad for you to study or exercise while you are eating, or right after eating? 2. How does overwork, or over-training, affect the heart? 3. What kind of play or exercise strengthens it? 4. How does good food help it? 5. What is the best way to avoid heart diseases, rheumatism, consumption, and pneumonia? 6. How does outdoor air help heart-action? 7. How do alcohol and tobacco injure the blood system and heart? 8. Why is alcohol particularly bad for underfed and overworked people? 9. At what two points is the blood system most likely to give way? 10. What may cause this breakage, or leakage? 11. What "catching" diseases often cause organic disease of the heart? 12. Why should heavy muscular work or strain be avoided after an attack of one of these diseases? 13. How may valvular heart trouble be remedied? 14. In what way are the nerve and blood systems connected? 15. What signal have we that we are beginning to over-exercise the heart? 16. What do we mean by "tobacco heart"? 17. Tell how to take care of the heart.

CHAPTER XIII

1. How long can an animal live without eating? 2. How long can an animal

live without breathing? 3. Why is your body like a sponge? 4. What are cells? 5. How do they get their food? 6. How many kinds of waste come from the body cells? 7. How is each kind carried away from the body? 8. What does the blood carry from the lungs to the body cells? 9. Why does it not carry air? 10. What process keeps your body warm? 11. What happens if the body cannot get oxygen? 12. How are the human lungs formed? 13. What is the windpipe? What are the bronchi? 14. Draw a picture of the lung-tree showing how the tubes branch. 15. What is at the end of each tiny branch? 16. How do the windpipe and the esophagus differ in form? 17. Why is the windpipe stiff? 18. In what four ways is the air you breathe out different from that which you took in? 19. Why does lime-water become milky when you breathe into it? 20. When you run, why do you breathe more quickly? Why does your heart beat faster? 21. How can you improve your "wind"? 22. In fever, why do you breathe more rapidly? 23. How do the ribs and muscles help in breathing?

CHAPTER XIV

1. Why is "caged air" dangerous? 2. How is outdoor air kept clean and pure? 3. What is air made of? 4. In what ways do people poison the air? 5. How do plants help to clean the air? 6. What is the best way to ventilate a room? Why? 7. Why do you have recess? 8. How does impure air make children look and feel? 9. Why is an open fire not the best means of heating and ventilating? 10. See if the room you are now in is properly ventilated. Why, or why not? 11. What are disease germs? 12. Why is dusty air unwholesome? 13. What is the safest way to clean a room? 14. Name three groups of disease germs that float in the air. 15. Name three ways in which you can protect yourself against these germs. 16. What is a cold? 17. What is the best way to cure a cold? 18. How can you prevent colds? 19. What causes consumption (tuberculosis of the lungs)? 20. Does the tubercle bacillus attack other parts of the body? 21. Why should a consumptive hold a cloth before his face when coughing? 22. Why should his sputum be burned? 23. Why should he go to a camp or sanatorium? Give two reasons. 24. About how much money could this country afford to spend in fighting consumption? Why? 25. Why need we no longer dread it as people did twenty-five years ago? 26. What methods are used in curing the disease? 27. What methods are used for preventing it? 28. Give two reasons why spitting should be prohibited. 29. What will fresh-air and sunlight do to the disease germs in the dust? 30. What do we know about the germs of pneumonia? 31. Do those who use alcohol stand a good chance

in fighting pneumonia? 32. How may pneumonia be prevented?

CHAPTER XV

1. Why is the skin so important? 2. Name some of the things that it does. 3. How many layers has it? Describe each. 4. What glands are found in the skin? 5. What is sweat, or perspiration, and from what does it come? 6. Why should clothing be porous? 7. Why should clothing be frequently washed? 8. Describe a hair gland and its muscles. 9. Describe the process of "nail-making." 10. Is there any process like this among the lower animals? 11. Why do we need nails? 12. What causes the white crescent on the nail? 13. Explain how the skin is a heat regulator. 14. What is the "normal temperature" of the body? 15. How does perspiring affect the heat of the body? 16. What are the "nerve buds" or "bulbs"? 17. Name four things that they do.

CHAPTER XVI

1. What are the uses of the skin to the rest of the body? 2. In what two ways does the skin clean itself? 3. What should we specially avoid in washing or scrubbing the skin? 4. What are the characteristics of a good soap? 5. What are the dangers of a poor soap? 6. What are the advantages of cold water in bathing? 7. How often should hot baths be taken and why? 8. On what parts of the body should soap be most freely used? 9. What is the best way of keeping the hair and scalp healthy? 10. Why is this important? 11. Why should hair tonics be let alone? 12. What causes dandruff? 13. How should the nails be trimmed and cleaned? 14. What should be done to the nail-fold? 15. Why is dirt under the nails sodangerous? 16. What qualities should a good garment possess as to shape, fit, and texture? 17. What are the advantages and disadvantages of wool? 18. What are the advantages and disadvantages of cotton? 19. Why are furs unwholesome? 20. What is the best possible material for an undergarment? 21. What are some of the causes of diseases of the skin? 22. What is the cause of sunburn and freckles? 23. What makes a good complexion? 24. What is a corn? What causes it?

CHAPTER XVII

1. Name four processes that take place in the living body. 2. What two kinds of waste do these processes cause? 3. What is the name of the "body smoke"?

4. How is the body smoke carried away? 5. What do the terms "soluble" and "insoluble" waste mean? 6. How does the insoluble waste leave the body? 7. By what path does the soluble waste leave the body? 8. How many times in an hour is all the blood in the body pumped through the liver, kidneys, and skin? 9, Why is this done? 10. Why is the blood from the food tube sent to the liver directly, instead of by way of the heart? 11. Why is the liver such a large organ? 12. What does the liver do to the blood? 13. What is the bile duct? 14. What is the bile? 15. What is the gall bladder? 16. What do the terms "bilious" and "jaundiced" mean? 17. What effect does alcohol have upon the liver?

CHAPTER XVIII

1. What is muscle? How much of your body weight is made up of the muscles? 2. What two kinds of muscles are there? 3. How do muscles change in shape? 4. What do we mean by voluntary and involuntary muscles, and how do they differ in form and location? 5. Describe the way in which the body muscles are arranged. What kind of actions do they perform? 6. What exercise is good for the muscles over the abdomen? for the muscles of the back? 7. What muscles are we using when we "bat" or "serve" in ball and tennis? 8. How do the muscles of the limbs act for you? 9. Where are the biceps and triceps muscles? Explain their use. 10. What are tendons? What is their use (function)? 11. How is your arm fastened to your body? 12. Describe the arrangement of the muscles in the lower limb. Why are they larger than the arm-muscles? 13. How does exercising the muscles give you an appetite? What else does it do? 14. Why do you naturally love to play? 15. Why is muscular exercise in the open air important in education?

CHAPTER XIX

1. What are the bones? 2. Make a rough sketch of the human skeleton. 3. In what sense are the bones the tools of the muscles? 4. How are the bones of the skull arranged? 5. Give two functions (uses) of the spinal column (back bone). 6. What bones and tendons do you use when you stand on tip-toe? 7. How are the limbs fastened to the body and back bone? 8. Why is the collar-bone more likely to be broken than some of the other bones? 9. How are the joints formed? 10. What is cartilage? 11. How does it help in making the two kinds of joints we find in the body? 12. Is there any arrangement for oiling the

joints? If so, what is it? 13. When you soak a bone in weak acid, what happens? What does this prove? 14. What causes disease or deformity of the bones?

CHAPTER XX

1. Why do we need a system of nerves? 2. What do we mean by motor nerves? by sensory nerves? 3. How is the central system like a telephone office? 4. What does the word ganglion mean to you? 5. What are the ganglions (ganglia) for? 6. Is the brain a ganglion? 7. Give a rough idea of the structure of the brain, and name its parts or divisions. 8. What does each one of these divisions do? 9. What is the result of injury to any one of these parts? Give an instance. 10. Where do we find the gray matter in the nervous system? 11. What is the white matter and what does it do? 12. When the thumb is paralyzed, what do we know about the brain? 13. Where in the body do we really smell, hear, and see? 14. What do we know about the speech centre? 15. Draw a picture of the spinal cord and its branches. 16. Of what use are the ganglia (gray matter) in the spinal cord? Give an example. 17. Why is it that some children can't help wriggling when tickled? 18. Why is the medulla such an important part of the nervous system? 19. When you touch a hot lamp chimney, what happens in your nervous system? 20. Suppose you had seen some tempting fruit, what would have happened in your nervous system and in your digestive system? 21. What does the brain do with the messages from the eyes, ears, and nose? 22. How does the message-and-answer system protect the body? 23. How does it help us to gain knowledge? 24. Why is it that when two people look at the same thing at the same time they may have very different ideas of what it is?

CHAPTER XXI

1. Describe the arches of the feet and tell what they are for. 2. Describe the kind of shoe you ought to wear. 3. Do you grow while asleep? 4. How much sleep do you need? 5. Are there many diseases of the muscles and bones? 6. How does nature repair a broken bone? 7. What causes most of the diseases of bones? 8. What is a slouching gait due to? 9. What is the cause of headache? 10. How should headache be regarded and treated? 11. What are the dangers of taking patent or unknown medicines? 12. What do most patent medicines contain? 13. Are the nerves resistant to disease, or specially

subject to its attack? 14. What causes many of the diseases of the nerves? 15. Name some poisons that injure the nerves? 16. How may diphtheria affect the nerves? 17. What does alcohol do to the nervous system? 18. Does our modern method of life tend to cause or to cure nervous diseases and insanity? Why?

CHAPTER XXII

1. How much of the body will muscular exercise develop? 2. Why should exercise and play be in the open air? 3. What is fatigue and what does it mean? 4. Name some games that are good exercise for the body and tell why they are so. 5. Why do marching and singing and drawing alternating with your other lessons, help you to grow? 6. Is playing a waste of time? Why? 7. How much exercise a day does a grown man or woman need? 8. How should this exercise be taken? 9. What senses and powers does base-ball develop? 10. In what respects is your progress in school work like your progress in learning to play games well? 11. What are good games for girls? 12. Why have we less sickness in summer than in winter? 13. Why is gardening a valuable occupation? 14. When should we do our hardest studying? 15. What is the best and most successful way to study? 16. How can you make school work as enjoyable as play? 17. What are your duties to-day? Plan the best way to do them so that you can also take exercise and rest and time for meals. Write this plan in the form of a day's programme.

CHAPTER XXIII

1. What is the "Lookout Department" of the body, and how is the work of this department distributed among the members? 2. Describe the inside structure of the nose. 3. In what sense is the nose like a radiator? 4. What are the cilia for? 5. How does the nose dispose of dust and lint? 6. What causes catarrh and colds? 7. Where is the sense of smell located? 8. When you have a cold, why do you often lose your sense of smell? of taste? 9. How do you tell the difference in flavor between an apple and an onion? 10. What does the tongue do? 11. What are the only tastes perceived in the mouth? 12. What does a coated tongue mean? 13. Is the sense of taste a safe guide in choosing foods? Why? 14. What are adenoids? What trouble do they cause? How can they be cured? 15. How does the eye help to choose food? 16. Name and describe the parts of the face around the eye. 17. Of what use is

each? 18. How does the tear gland act? 19. What is the retina? the pupil? the iris? What is each for? 20. What do we mean by bringing the rays of light to a focus? How can you illustrate this by a burning glass? 21. When do eyes need glasses? 22. How can the eye change the form of its lens for near and for far sight? What is this action called? 23. Why do children born deaf become dumb? 24. Where do we find the key-board of hearing? Why do we call it the cochlea? 25. Draw a picture showing the position of the drum, "hammer," "anvil," "stirrup," and cochlea. 26. What has happened in your inner ear when something in your ear goes "pop"? 27. Why does a cold sometimes make you deaf? 28. Why do we have wax in the outer ear? What is the German proverb about cleaning the ear? 29. What is our "sixth sense"? Where do we find its organ located? What is it like?

CHAPTER XXIV

1. How is the voice a waste product? 2. What are the conditions required to make a good voice? 3. Are great singers usually strong? Why? 4. How was the windpipe made into the voice box? 5. Describe the vocal bands or cords. 6. How do they act in making voice sounds? when we breathe? 7. How do catarrh and adenoids affect the voice? 8. How is the voice box like a violin? 9. What part of the violin has most to do with the quality of the sound? How does this apply to the human voice? 10. What do the throat, the mouth, and the nose have to do with voice training? 11. What is one of the commonest causes of a poor voice? 12. How can you prove this? 13. What are spoken words? 14. How is a good, clear, distinct voice of value? 15. How can you build up a strong, clear, useful voice?

CHAPTER XXV

1. Give four reasons why the teeth are important. 2. To take proper care of the teeth, what other parts of the mouth need attention? 3. Draw a picture of a tooth and label the crown, the enamel, the root, the pulp. 4. Name the different teeth, making diagrams of the upper and lower jaws and tell how each kind of tooth is used. 5. Compare your own teeth with those of a dog, a sheep, and a squirrel and explain the difference in use. 6. In what order did your teeth appear in your mouth? 7. What are the milk-teeth? 8. How many teeth have you? Have any been pulled? 9. Will you have any more later? 10. Name three things to be remembered in exercising the teeth. 11. What is the

best method to keep the teeth and gums clean? 12. Why are "gritty" tooth-powders bad for the teeth? 13. Are antiseptics good for them? 14. Why are dirty teeth a very common cause of disease in the body? 15. (Exercise) Write a letter to your teacher telling how you have been taking care of your teeth in the past, and how you purpose to do it in the future.

CHAPTER XXVI

1. How may "catching" diseases be prevented? 2. What are disease germs, and how are they named? 3. How do disease germs grow? 4. Why should patients with the "diseases of childhood" be placed in quarantine. 5. What causes a cold? How should you take care of one? Why keep away from other people? 6. When and how did we find that diphtheria was due to germs? 7. Explain how "antitoxin" prevents it. 8. How much has the death rate in diphtheria been lowered? 9. Name the diseases for which we now have vaccines and antitoxins. How do we grow them? 10. Tell the story about Dr. Jenner and the milkmaids. 11. What good has his discovery done? 12. Explain why vaccination will cure as well as prevent smallpox. 13. What is quinine, and where does it get its name? 14. Who discovered the germ of malaria? Is it a plant or an animal? 15. What do we know about the connection between mosquitoes and malaria? 16. What is a quick way of killing the mosquito? 17. How does draining fields prevent malaria? Why is malaria not so common now as in pioneer days? 18. Why do we need disinfectants? Name some, and describe how they are used. 19. What is the best one in most cases? Why? In what ways may it be used? 20. How do the bacteria of the soil "feed" the green plants? 21. Explain why a crop of clover will enrich the soil. What other plants also do the same thing? 22. Name some other harmless bacteria. 23. Why ought one to wash the hands before eating? 24. Is it possible to kill all house flies? Why ought we to try to? How can it be done? 25. What do we find in dust? 26. What good does it do to sprinkle streets? 27. What is the best way to clean house?

CHAPTER XXVII

1. What is the best insurance against accidents? 2. Why do most cuts and scratches heal quickly, while some others do not? 3. What kind of dirt is dangerous to wounds? 4. If your knife should slip and cut you, how ought you to take care of the cut? 5. If you know the knife is dirty, what is the proper

treatment? 6. Is "sticking-plaster" good for a wound? Why not? 7. Why does absorbent cotton make a good dressing? 8. Give two reasons why doctors can perform surgical operations now much more safely than some years ago. 9. Why must surgeons and nurses keep themselves and their patients perfectly clean? 10. What difference has this cleanliness made in the saving of life? 11. What is the treatment for bruises? Why are they not so dangerous as cuts? 12. What are boils and carbuncles? 13. How do we clean and heal them? 14. Where blood comes in spurts from a cut, what does this mean? 15. How does the blood itself protect us against infection in wounds? 16. If the wound is very deep, how can you check the bleeding? 17. Why should the tight bandage be slightly loosened in half an hour after it has been applied? 18. Why is it that we do not need to clean a burn? 19. Why is it wise to keep the air from a burn? How may it be done? 20. Why must the dressings be perfectly clean? 21. Why do we need a doctor in the case of a broken bone? 22. If you can't get a doctor, what is to be done? 23. What is a sprain? Tell how to bathe and bandage it. 24. In the case of swallowing poison, why should one drink warm water? 25. What else should be done? 26. What should be given when lye has been swallowed? 27. What is the important thing to remember in any such case? 28. If you fall into deep water, what four things should you remember? 29. Explain carefully just how to revive a person who has been under water. 30. What is the main purpose of this method?

GLOSSARY

OF IMPORTANT TERMS USED IN THE BOOK

[Transcriber's note: In the following section vowels are transcribed as: [)vowel] with breve [=vowel] with macron [.vowel] with dot above]

I. RELATING TO THE BODY AS A WHOLE

Ab'do men (or [)a]b d[=o]'m[)e]n). The cavity of the trunk immediately below the diaphragm.

Car'ti lage. Tough, elastic tissue, generally more or less fibrous; called also gristle (gr[)i]s'l).

Cell. The simplest form of living matter, with power to grow, develop, reproduce itself, and, with others of its kind, build up a living fabric.

Di'a phragm (d[=i]'[.a] fr[)a]m). The muscular membrane that separates the thorax from the abdomen.

Duct. A tube through which fluid from a gland is conveyed.

Fa tigue' (f[.a] t[=e]g'). A condition in which the body cells are worn out faster than they are built up, so that waste matter accumulates in the body and poisons it.

Germ. The simplest form of life, from which a living organism develops.

Gland. A part, or organ, that has the power of making a secretion, peculiar to itself. A gland may be a simple pocket, or follicle, as is an oil gland of the skin, or it may be an aggregate of such glands, as is the liver.

Or'gan. Any part, or member, that has some specific function, or duty, by which some one of the body's activities is carried on; for example, the eye is the organ of vision, the liver is one of the organs of digestion.

Tho'rax. The cavity of the trunk immediately above the diaphragm.

Tis'sue (t[)i]sh'[=u]). A fabric, or texture, composed of cells and cell-products of one kind; as, for example, nervous tissue, muscular tissue, fatty tissue.

Se cre'tion. A substance made from the blood, the special character of which depends upon the kind of gland that makes, or secretes, it.

II. RELATING TO THE DIGESTIVE SYSTEM

Al i men'ta ry ca nal'. The food tube, or digestive tube, extending from lips and nose to the end of the rectum, with its various branches and attachments.

Bile. A yellow, bitter, alkaline liquid secreted by the liver, and especially valuable in the digestion of fats; sometimes called gall.

Co'lon. The large intestine.

Di ges'tion. The process in the body by which food is changed to the form in which it can pass from the alimentary canal to the blood vessels and lymphatics.

Di ges'tive sys'tem. The alimentary canal with all its branches and appendages; that is, all the organs that directly take part in the process of digestion.

E soph'a gus. The tube through which food and drink pass from the pharynx to the stomach; called also the gul'let.

Gall blad'der. The bile bladder; the sac, or reservoir, lying on the under side of the liver, in which the bile is received from the liver, and in which it is retained until discharged through the gall duct into the small intestine.

Gas'tric juice. The digestive liquid secreted by the glands of the stomach (pep'tic glands); it contains pepsin, acid, and ferments; called also peptic juice.

In tes'tine. The last part of the alimentary canal, extending from the pylorus. Its length is five or six times that of the body. The greater part of its length is called the small intestine in distinction from the remaining part, which, though much shorter, is larger in diameter, and is called the large intestine or co'lon. The intestine as a whole is sometimes called the bow'el.

Liv'er. The large gland that secretes bile and is active in changing or killing harmful substances; located in the upper part of the abdominal cavity, on the right side, and folds over on the pyloric end of the stomach.

Lym phat'ics. Small transparent tubes running through the various tissues, and containing a colorless fluid somewhat thinner than blood, called lymph. This fluid is composed of the leakage from the arteries and of wastes from the tissues, which are being carried to a larger lymph duct to be emptied into one of the larger veins. The lymphatics in the wall of the intestine take up some of the digested food from the cells and pass it on through the lymph glands of the abdomen to the lymph duct which empties into a vein near the heart.

Mas ti ca'tion. The process of grinding, or chewing, food in the mouth.

Mes'en ter y. The tissue (part of the peritoneum) which is attached to the intestine and, for a few inches, to the spinal column, to hold the coils of the intestine in place.

Mu'cous mem'brane. The lining membrane, or tissue, of the entire alimentary canal. It is very complex in structure, has different characteristics in different areas, and contains nerves, blood vessels, lymphatics, and in various parts special structures such as glands. It secretes mucous. It is continuous with the outside skin of the body, as may be seen at the lips.

Pan'cre as. The gland that secretes the pancreatic juice; located in the abdominal cavity near the stomach.

Pan cre at'ic juice. An alkaline digestive juice poured by the pancreas into the small intestine; especially valuable in the digestion of starches, fats, and proteins.

Per i to ne'um. The membrane lining the abdominal cavity and enfolding its organs.

Phar'ynx. The passage between the nasal passages and the esophagus: the throat.

Py lor'us. (1) The opening from the stomach into the small intestine. (2) The fold of mucous membrane, containing muscle fibres, that helps to regulate the passage of food through the pyloric opening.

Sa li'va. The digestive secretion in the mouth, consisting of the secretion of the salivary glands and the secretion of the mucous membrane of the mouth.

Stom'ach. The pouch-like enlargement of the alimentary canal, lying in the upper part of the abdominal cavity, and slightly to the left, between the esophagus and the small intestine.

III. RELATING TO FOOD AND DRINK

Ac'id ([)a]s'[)i]d). A substance (usually sour tasting) that has, among other properties, the power of combining with an alkali in such a way that both substances lose their peculiar characteristics and form a salt.

Al'co hol. A colorless liquid formed by the fermentation of starch-sugars or certain other substances, which is highly inflammable and burns without smoke or waste; it is a stimulant and an antiseptic.

Al'ka li. A substance that has, among other properties, the power of neutralizing acids and forming salts with them. (See Acid.)

Car'bo hy'drates. Plant or animal substances composed of carbon, hydrogen, and oxygen. (Called also starch-sugars.)

Chlo'ro phyll. The green coloring matter of plants, formed by the action of sunlight on the plant cells. It is a necessary part of the plant's digestive system, since without it the plant could not break up the carbon dioxid of the air into the carbon which it uses in preparing its starch food, and the oxygen which it gives off as waste.

Fer men ta'tion. A chemical change in plant or animal substance, produced usually by the action of bacteria, in the process of which the substance is broken up (decomposed), and new substances are formed.

Nar cot'ic. Any substance that blunts the senses, or the body's sensibility to pain or discomfort.

Ni'tro gen. A tasteless, odorless, colorless gas, forming nearly four-fifths of the earth's atmosphere; and constituting a necessary part of every plant and animal tissue.

Pro'te ins. Foods containing a large amount of nitrogen; such as meat, fish, milk, egg, peas, beans.

IV. RELATING TO THE BLOOD AND THE CIRCULATORY SYSTEM

A or'ta. The main artery of the body; it leads out from the left ventricle of the heart, carrying arterialized blood (blood that has been acted upon by oxygen) to all parts of the body except the lungs.

Ar'te ries. The blood vessels and their branches that carry blood from the heart to all parts of the body. The pul'mon a ry artery carries impure (ve'nous) blood to the lungs.

Au'ri cles (?r[)i] klz). The two chambers of the heart that receive blood from the veins.

Cap'il la ries. The minute blood vessels which form a network between the ends of the arteries and the beginnings of the veins.

Cir cu la'tion. The passage of the blood from the heart into the arteries, and from them through the capillaries into the veins, and through the veins back into the heart.

Cor'pus cles (cor'p[)u]s'lz). Minute jelly-like disks or cells. These are of two kinds, red and white, the red (the oxygen carriers) being about 350 times as many as the white, and giving the blood its color.

Heart. A muscle-sac located in the thorax between the lungs, its lower point, or a'pex, being tilted somewhat to the left; the centre and force-pump of the circulatory system.

Ox i da'tion. Combining with oxygen.

Ox'y gen. A colorless, odorless, tasteless gas, which forms about one-fifth of the earth's atmosphere. It is found in all animal and vegetable tissues. When it combines with other substances, a certain amount of heat is produced; and if the process is sufficiently rapid, a flame is seen.

Pulse. The regularly recurring enlargement of an artery, caused by the increased blood flow following each contraction of the ventricle of the heart.

Veins. The blood vessels and their branches through which blood flows from all parts of the body back to the heart. All the veins except the pulmonary veins carry impure (venous) blood; the pulmonary veins carry arterialized (oxidated) blood from the lungs. Ve'na ca'va. Either of the two large veins discharging into the right auricle of the heart. Por'tal vein. The large, short vein that drains the liver and adjacent parts.

Ven'tri cles. The two chambers of the heart that receive blood from the auricles and force it into the arteries.

V. RELATING TO THE RESPIRATORY SYSTEM AND ORGANS OF EXCRETION

Al ve'o li ([)a]l v[=e]'o l[=i]). (Plural of alveolus). Air cells. The cells, or cavities, that line the air passages and air sacs at the ends of the bronchial tubes.

Breath. Air taken in or sent out in respiration; that breathed out containing carbon dioxid, watery vapor, and various impurities.

Bron'chi (br[)o]n'k[=i]). (Plural of bronchus). The two main branches of the trachea. These branch into numerous smaller branches, called the bron'chi al tubes.

Car'bon di ox'id. A gas formed of carbon and oxygen; colorless and odorless; has a somewhat acid taste, and is used for aerating soda water and other beverages; is present naturally in mineral and spring waters. It is present largely in the fissures of the earth and makes the choke-damp of mines. Called also car bon'ic acid.

Ep i glot'tis. The valve-like cover that prevents food and drink from entering the larynx.

Ex cre'tion. A waste substance thrown out, or rejected, from the system; for example, carbon dioxid, sweat, ur'ine, the fe'ces.

Lar'ynx. The enlargement of the windpipe, near its upper end, across which are stretched the vocal cords.

Lungs. Two spongy organs in the thorax, entered by the bronchi with their bronchial tubes; they contain in the walls of their air cells the capillaries through which the blood passes from the branches of the pulmonary artery to the branches of the pulmonary veins.

Rec'tum. The lowest and last section of the alimentary canal, being the discharge pipe of the large intestine, and excreting the solid wastes in the form of the feces.

Res pi ra'tion. Breathing; the action of the body by which carbon dioxid is given off from the blood and a corresponding amount of oxygen is absorbed into the blood.

Skin. The continuous outer covering of the body, in the deeper layer (der'ma) of which are located the sweat glands, which secrete sweat (a watery, oily substance containing impurities from the blood) and excrete it through the sweat ducts and their openings (pores) in the surface of the skin.

Tra'che a (or tr[=a] ch[=e]' [.a]). The windpipe between the larynx and the bronchi.

U'ri na ry system. The organs concerned in the secretion and discharge of urine: the kid'neys (two glands in the abdominal cavity, back of the peritoneum, which receive wastes from the blood, and excrete them as urine), the u re'ters (ducts through which the urine flows from the kidneys to the bladder), the blad'der (an elastic muscle-sac in which the urine is retained until discharged from the body).

VI. RELATING TO THE NERVOUS AND MOTOR SYSTEMS

Brain. The soft mass of nerve tissue filling the upper cavity of the skull. Its cellular tissue is gray, and its fibrous tissue white. With the spinal cord it controls all the sensory and motor activities of the body.

Cer e bel'lum. The part of the brain lying below the hind part of the cerebrum.

Cer'e brum. The upper or fore part of the brain; it is divided by a deep fissure into two hemispheres, its cor'tex (surface) lies in many con vo lu'tions (folds), and its fibres run down into the spinal cord. In this part of the brain are the centres, or controlling nerve cells, of the senses and most of our conscious activities.

Gang'li a (g[)a]ng'l[)i] [.a]). (Plural of ganglion). Nerve knots, or groupings of nerve cells, forming an enlargement in the course of a nerve.

Me dul'la. A portion of the brain forming an enlargement at the top of the spinal cord and being continuous with it; the channel between the brain and the other parts of the nervous system.

Muscle (mus'l). A kind of animal tissue that consists of fibres that have the power of contracting when properly stimulated. A bundle of muscle fibres, called a muscle, is usually attached to the part to be moved by a ten'don, or sinew. Muscles causing bones to bend are termed flex'ors; those causing them to straighten, ex ten'sors. The movements of muscles may be voluntary (controlled by the will), or involuntary (made without conscious exercise of the will).

Nerve. A fibre of nerve tissue, or a bundle of such fibres, connecting nerve ganglia with each other or with some terminal nerve organ. Nerves running inward toward the spinal cord and the brain are called sen'so ry nerves; those from the brain and spinal cord outward, mo'tor nerves.

Nerv'ous system. The nerve centres with the sensory and motor nerves and the organs of sense.

Neu'rons. The cells of the spinal cord and the brain.

Re'flex. A simple action of the nervous system, in which a stimulus is carried along sensory nerves to a nerve centre, and from which an answering stimulus is sent along motor nerves to call into play the activity of some organ, without consciousness, or without direct effort of the will.

Spi'nal cord. The soft nerve tissue that extends from the medulla almost to the end of the spinal column, being encased by it. It controls most of the reflex actions of the body.

Stim'u lus. Anything that starts an activity in the tissues on which it acts; for example, light is a stimulus to the nerve tissues of the eye.

###